常见心血管病

调养功法

彭锐 著

SPM 南方传媒 | 广东科技出版社
全国优秀出版社

· 广 州 ·

图书在版编目（CIP）数据

常见心血管病调养功法 / 彭锐著. —广州：广东科技出版社，
2023.12

ISBN 978-7-5359-8195-0

Ⅰ.①常⋯ Ⅱ.①彭⋯ Ⅲ.①心脏血管疾病 – 中医治疗
法 Ⅳ.①R259.4

中国国家版本馆CIP数据核字（2023）第237245号

常见心血管病调养功法
Changjian Xinxueguanbing Tiaoyang Gongfa

出 版 人：严奉强
责任编辑：李 婷 黄豪杰
装帧设计：友间文化
责任校对：陈 静
责任印制：彭海波
出版发行：广东科技出版社
（广州市环市东路水荫路11号 邮政编码：510075）
销售热线：020-37607413
https://www.gdstp.com.cn
E-mail：gdkjbw@nfcb.com.cn
经 销：广东新华发行集团股份有限公司
印 刷：广州一龙印刷有限公司
（广州市增城区荔新九路43号 邮政编码：511340）
规 格：890 mm×1 240 mm 1/32 印张4.75 字数115千
版 次：2023年12月第1版
2023年12月第1次印刷
定 价：39.80元

作者
简介

现任广州中医药大学顺德医院副院长，硕士研究生导师，国医大师邓铁涛学术继承人，广东省高等学校中青年教师国内访问学者（导师张伯礼院士），广东省名中医继承人，广东省社区卫生学会中医药与适宜技术分会副会长，香港大学校外评审主任。

临床擅长运用体质学说辨证治疗心血管病、肺系病症、脾胃病及内科疑难杂症，师从国医大师邓铁涛、全国名老中医张伯礼院士、广东省名中医吴伟和汤水福，精于临床辨证，病机把握准确，尤其擅长中西医结合治疗心脑血管疾病（高血压、冠心病、双心疾病、心力衰竭、肾衰竭等），常年习练"邓氏八段锦"、易筋经等养生功法，对养生保健有独到的观点和研究。

彭 锐

医学博士　副教授
副主任中医师

序言

Preface

　　彭锐博士是一位医术精湛的医生，现任广州中医药大学顺德医院副院长，硕士研究生导师，以中西医结合治疗心脑血管疾病见长。其人文学科功底深厚，早在2009年9月28日晚上广州中医药大学大学城校区，万名青年学子举行庆祝中华人民共和国成立60周年大型文艺晚会上，朗诵《苍生大医》，描述国医大师邓铁涛教授岁月如歌的一生，全场欢声雷动，掀起晚会高潮，令笔者难以忘怀。今读其著述《常见心血管病调养功法》，又令笔者耳目一新，如白居易《修香山寺记》："关塞之气色，龙潭之景象，香山之泉石，石楼之风月，与往来者耳目一时而新。"该书不仅是用文字表述，而且作者身体力行演练调养功法，图文并茂，内容包括高血压及失眠调治（降压助眠功法）、心功能不全调治（补气强身功法）、眩晕调治（整脊松项功法）三部分，以及英文对照与常见心血管病相关科普知识等，既专业严谨又通俗易懂，想来必受广大读者欢迎。

　　与彭锐博士相识久矣，他是"邓氏八段锦"第三代（邓铁涛→邓中光→彭锐）学术传承人，三代人各自演练"邓氏八段锦"，在电视屏幕与各大中医院播放，制作音像光碟广泛传播，造福民众病患，从学者众，受益者无数。邓铁涛，国医大师；邓中光，广东省名中医；彭锐虽年轻也小有名气，一脉相承。例如书中"降压助眠功法"共有九个招式：第一式揉按百会脑窍清，第二式点压风池耳目明，第三式点揉迎香鼻窍通，第四式顺捋太阳头痛宁，第五式摩捋阳经肢轻缓，第六式揉按膻中心脉畅，第七式捋按肾俞身常暖，第八式点压脾肾脑髓充，第九式点按太冲气自安。其所采用的调养功法传承了邓铁涛教授应用外治法降压调心助眠的学术经验。

养生保健功法源自古代中医导引术，源远流长。如长沙马王堆出土文物西汉彩绘帛书《导引图》中有"坐引八维"（坐立导引四面八方）图，后人注解"引八维以自道（导）分，含沉瀣以长生"。又如东汉华佗创编的"五禽戏"，"晓养性之术，时人以为年且百岁而貌有壮容"。它们是当代医疗保健功法的学术源泉及理论依据。作为当代中医，只会单纯处方用药诊治疾病是远远不够的，君不见国医大师邓铁涛教授"攒拳怒目增气力"的英姿。彭锐博士在临床实践中体会到心血管病的康养调理很重要，拜学名师如张伯礼院士、广东省名中医吴伟和汤水福等，勤求古训、博采众方，把前人及老师学术经验逐步凝练成著作。《常见心血管病调养功法》就是彭锐博士传承创新成果之载体，读后深有感触，故乐为之序。

刘小斌　广州中医药大学教授，博士研究生导师
全国老中医药专家学术经验继承工作指导老师
2023年3月23日

前言

Preface

  心血管病是当今社会人类健康的第一杀手，如今针对心血管病的治疗方案也越来越丰富，但是作为心血管医生的我，看到的现状是，高血压患者越来越多、越来越年轻化，心脏支架手术越来越多，失眠焦虑患者不断增加，颈椎病、腰椎病发病率居高不下，国家医保的支出越来越多，到底是什么原因造成了这种现状呢？

  排在首位的原因我认为当数人们的健康意识和科学观念欠缺。当今社会信息爆炸，而这些信息良莠不齐，很多患者每天拿着错误的信息咨询我是不是可以照做，消耗了大量的时间和精力。能够正确认识常见心血管病，对常见心血管病的病因有一定了解，懂得一些正确的处理方法，这是我希望所有心血管病患者都能做到的。自己是自己最好的医生，基于这种原因，我编写了这部具有临床指导意义和价值的《常见心血管病调养功法》，其中对于常见心血管病，如高血压、心功能不全、眩晕等有针对性地编制了调养功法，并对这些常见病进行了科普。结合我多年的养生保健功法习练经验，这套功法对于日常保健、维持心血管健康有着积极的作用和意义，可以改善患者症状，起到保健和预防作用，如果能够配合药物和中医治疗，可以起到事半功倍的效果！本书使用中英双语对照的形式，可以让更广大的人群受益，也期望中医药知识能够更加广泛地传播到全世界。

"但愿世间无疾病，何惜架上药生尘"，"彭博士跟您说"丛书各个分册将陆续出版，内容包含各类疾病的保健、预防、中医药养生等知识，希望大家都能够享受健康快乐的人生！

本书的编写得到广州中医药大学刘小斌教授、广州中医药大学邓中光教授及其夫人陈安琳女士的大力支持和协助，本书的英文部分得到长春中医药大学宿哲骞教授的指导，广州中医药大学梁蕾、吴佩烨、赖思燃、周桂庭、张紫艳同学在排版、校正方面付出了辛勤劳动，在此表示衷心感谢。

彭锐

2023年3月28日

目 录
Contents

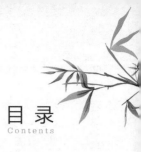

调养功法

高血压、失眠调治——降压助眠功法

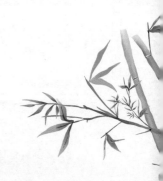

常见心血管病
相关科普知识

高血压

常见心血管病调养功法

心功能不全——心力衰竭

眩晕——颈椎病、腰椎病

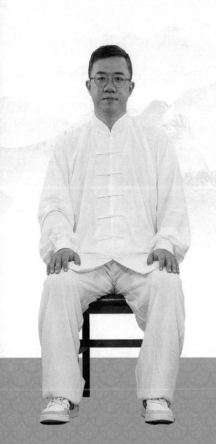

调养功法

高血压、失眠调治
——降压助眠功法

　　该功法以调节血压、改善睡眠为目的，根据中医学、针灸学、推拿学治疗疾病相关理论，结合彭博士多年的养生功法训练和研究创立。该功法以点、按、揉、压、捋、摩等按摩手法为基础，通过全身的综合运动带动气血的运行，达到调整阴阳、调畅气机、平肝潜阳、滋补肝肾的目的，从而治疗原发性高血压、失眠、头痛、头晕、抑郁焦虑、更年期综合征等相关疾病。

　　该功法将人体的作用位置分为了三大部分，分别是：头颈部、上肢躯干、下肢足部。以头颈部动作为主，辅以上肢躯干、下肢足部动作增强疗效。头颈部主要干预穴位为：百会、风池、头维、太阳、印堂、迎香及相关耳穴。上肢躯干主要干预穴位为：手三里、内关、合谷、膻中、带脉、肾俞、命门。下肢足部主要干预穴位为：血海、足三里、三阴交、太冲、涌泉。

功法顺序：从上到下，由左及右。

☯ 起势

采取靠坐式、站立式均可。以靠坐式为例。

⌇ 调身操作要点：全身放松，靠坐椅上，两目轻闭，舌抵上颚，两唇微闭，松肩垂肘；两足微分，与肩同宽。（图1）

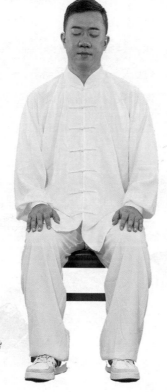

图1　起势

⌇ 调息操作要点：自然呼吸，心情平静，腹式呼吸。

⌇ 调心操作要点：精神放松，意守丹田，呼吸均匀。

常见心血管病调养功法

😊 第一式
揉按百会脑窍清

🍃 **调身操作要点**：左臂自左侧向上，左手小鱼际按于巅顶百会穴位置，力度均匀按压，共进行6次，之后按照逆时针顺序，用小鱼际揉按百会穴，共进行6次；之后换右手按照上述方法进行操作，注意右手按顺时针顺序揉按，均进行6次。左右手交替，每侧进行3遍，共6遍结束。（图2、图3）

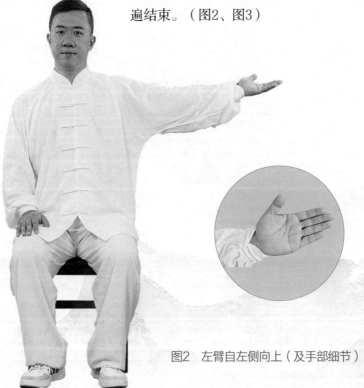

图2　左臂自左侧向上（及手部细节）

～ 调息操作要点：在按压百会穴过程中，按压时呼气，放松时吸气；揉按过程中平静呼吸，揉按速度不宜过快，呼吸一次，揉按一周。

～ 调心操作要点：心无旁骛，意守丹田。

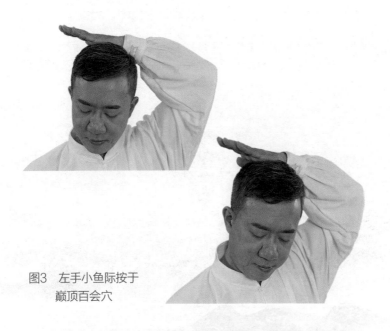

图3　左手小鱼际按于
　　　巅顶百会穴

～ 功法作用 ～

百会，别名"三阳五会"。属督脉，位于头部，前发际正中直上5寸。主治头痛、目眩、鼻塞、耳鸣、中风、失语等。按揉百会穴，可以起到开窍醒脑的作用，对于高血压患者常见的头晕、头痛等症状有良好的改善作用。

调养功法

☯ 第二式
点压风池耳目明

✍ 调身操作要点：双手自体侧向上抱头，双手拇指按于风池穴位置，其余手指虚掌置于头侧，力度适中均匀地按压风池穴，共进行6次，之后左手拇指逆时针、右手拇指顺时针对风池穴进行揉按，共6次，之后放松复位。如此循环4遍。（图4、图5）

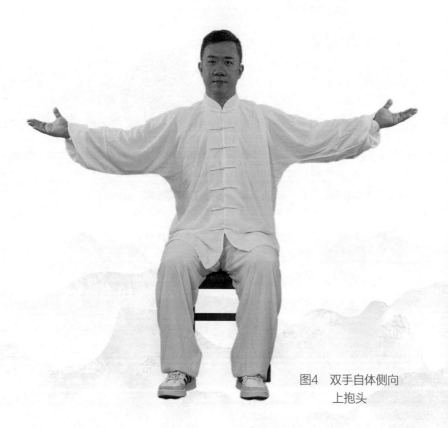

图4 双手自体侧向
上抱头

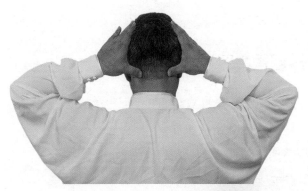

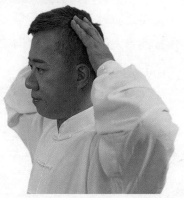

✎ 调息操作要点：

按压风池穴时呼气，放松时吸气；揉按过程中平静呼吸，揉按速度不宜过快，呼吸一次，揉按一周。

✎ 调心操作要点：

心无旁骛，意守丹田。

图5　双手拇指按于风池穴（正侧位演示）

✎ 功法作用 ✎

风池，属足少阳胆经，足少阳、阳维之会。在项部，当枕骨之下，与风府相平，胸锁乳突肌与斜方肌上端之间的凹陷处。主治头痛、头晕、伤风感冒、目赤肿痛、耳鸣、耳聋等。点压风池穴，可以起到平肝息风、通利官窍的作用，对于高血压和失眠患者的头部症状有明显的改善作用。

调养功法

☯ 第三式

点揉迎香鼻窍通

◠ 调身操作要点：双手呈"八"字状，双手食指从印堂穴滑下按压睛明穴、迎香穴，左、右手食指点按迎香穴6次，然后左手食指逆时针、右手食指顺时针揉按迎香穴6次。如此循环4遍。（图6～图8）

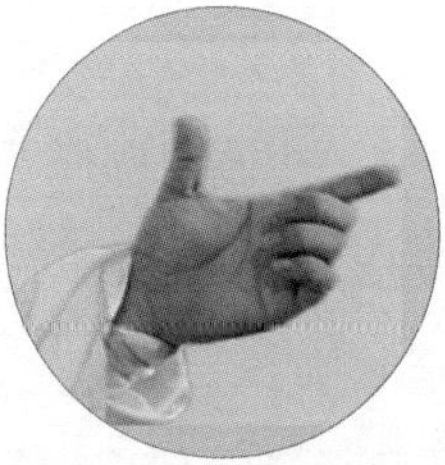

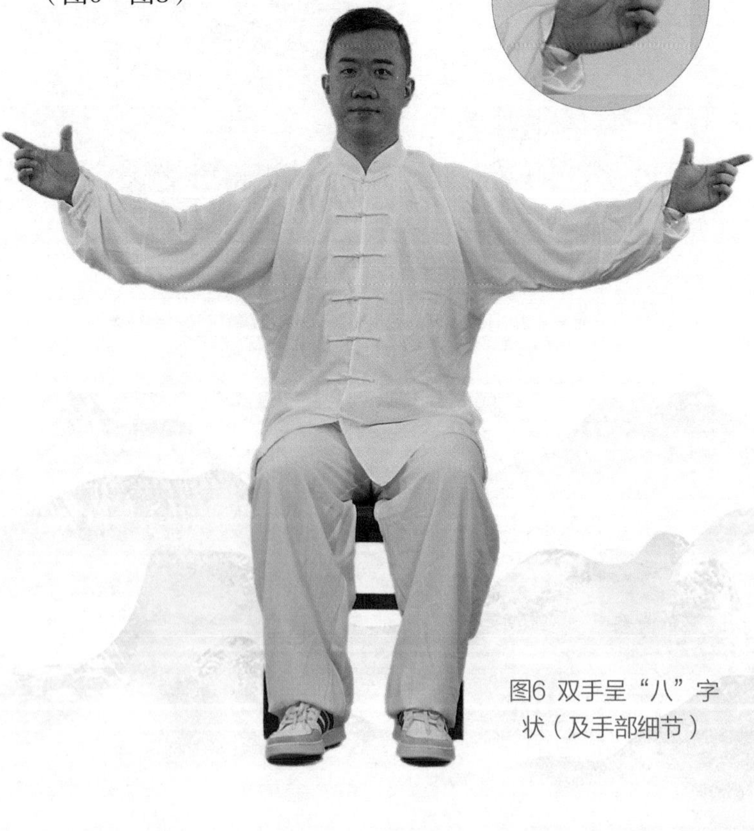

图6 双手呈"八"字状（及手部细节）

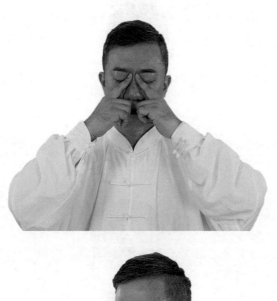

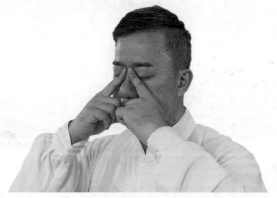

图7 食指从印堂穴滑下（正侧位演示）

    ⌒ 调息操作要点：整个过程平静呼吸，按压迎香穴时呼气，放松时吸气。

    ⌒ 调心操作要点：心无旁骛，意守丹田，想象一股气从印堂下移至鼻部。

调养功法

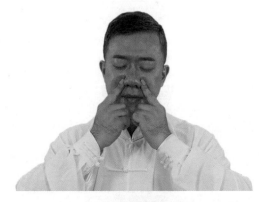

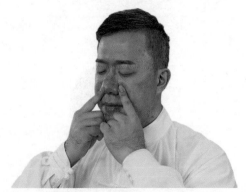

图8　食指滑下按压至迎香穴并点按（正侧位演示）

～ 功法作用 ～

迎香，属手阳明大肠经，此腧穴在鼻翼外缘中点旁，当鼻唇沟中；有疏散风热、通利鼻窍的作用；主要用于治疗鼻塞、衄衄、口歪等。按揉迎香穴可以通鼻窍、畅呼吸，对高血压、失眠患者的症状改善有良好的作用。

第四式
顺捋太阳头痛宁

🌀 调身操作要点：双手呈"剑指"，点按头维穴6次，之后缓慢滑下至太阳穴，左手逆时针、右手顺时针揉按太阳穴6次，之后手指滑下至耳尖，左、右手拇指与食指捏住耳廓外缘顺势下捋，在耳垂处捏压6次。如此循环4遍。（图9～图14）

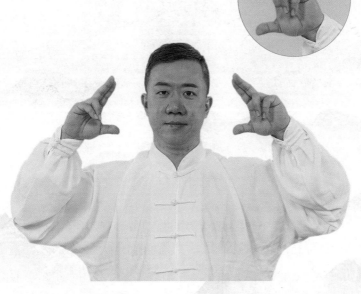

图9 双手呈"剑指"（及手部细节）

常见心血管病调养功法

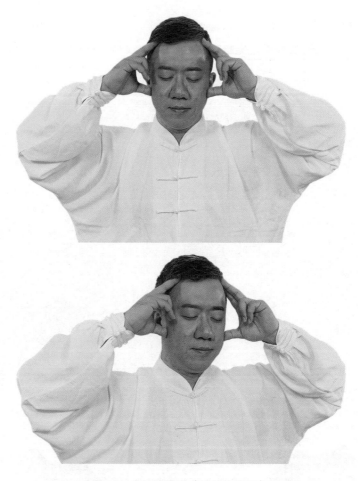

图10 点按头维穴（正侧位演示）

～ 调息操作要点：整个过程平静呼吸，在点按和揉按开始时呼气，放松时吸气，呼吸均匀舒缓。

～ 调心操作要点：心无旁骛，意守丹田，想象一股气从太阳穴下移至耳垂。

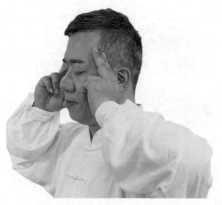

图11 手指滑下至
太阳穴并揉按

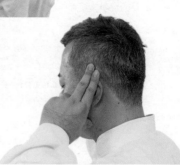

图12 手指继续滑下至耳尖

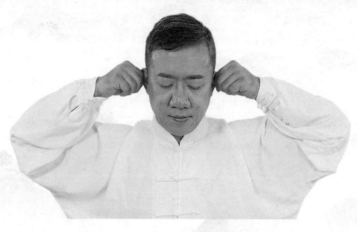

图13 拇指与食指捏住耳廓外缘顺势下捋

调养功法

常见心血管病调养功法

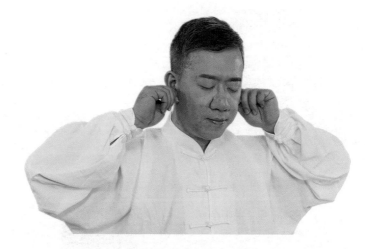

图14　顺势下捋至耳垂并捏压

❧ 功法作用 ❧

　　头维，为足阳明胃经腧穴，是足阳明胃经与足少阳胆经、阳维脉之交会穴。当额角发际上0.5寸，头正中线旁，距神庭4.5寸，在颞肌上缘帽状腱膜中；主治头痛、目眩、目痛、迎风流泪等。太阳，位于额部的两侧，眼眶的外上部，延伸至耳上沿；具有清热消肿、止痛舒络的功效，可以治疗偏头痛、目眩、口眼歪斜等。依顺序点按头维穴、揉按太阳穴、捏压耳垂，可以综合调节高血压及失眠患者的头部症状，如头痛、头晕、视物不清等。

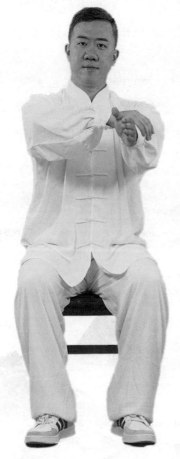

第五式
摩捋阳经肢轻缓

❧ 调身操作要点：左手平举于胸前，右手拇指按于左上臂内侧，其余四指位于左上臂外侧，右手拇指沿手厥阴心包经循行部位捋按，其余四指沿手阳明大肠经循行部位捋按，手三里穴按压3次，内关穴按压3次，合谷穴按压3次。左右手交替，共进行4遍。（图15～图17）

图15　左手平举于胸前，右手拇指按于左上臂内侧

调养功法

常见心血管病调养功法

〇 调息操作要点：整个过程平静呼吸，在向下捋按开始时呼气，放松时吸气，呼吸均匀舒缓。

〇 调心操作要点：心无旁骛，意守丹田，目视前方，想象有气从肩部沿上肢内外两侧向下运行至指尖。

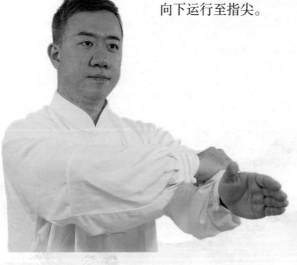

图16　手部沿经脉循行部位捋按并沿途按压手三里穴、内关穴

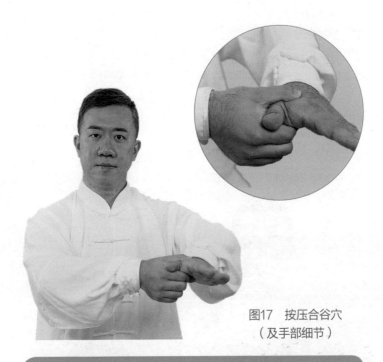

图17　按压合谷穴
（及手部细节）

　　手厥阴心包经经穴主要治疗心、胸、胃病，神志病及经脉循行部位的其他病症。治疗心、胸、胃病常用曲泽、郄门、间使、内关和大陵，治疗神志病常用间使、劳宫、中冲；内关有宣通三焦、醒脑开窍、行气止痛的功效，天池以治疗胸胁痛、心肺病为主。手阳明大肠经本经腧穴主要治疗头面、五官、咽喉病，神志病，热病及经脉循行部位的其他病症。同时掐按表里经，可以全方位刺激相应经穴，对于高血压和失眠患者心、胸部的不适，具有很好的症状改善作用。

调养功法

常见心血管病调养功法

🌓 第六式
揉按膻中心脉畅

  🌊 调身操作要点：左手小鱼际置于膻中穴位置，按压6次，然后逆时针揉按6次。左右手交替，共进行4遍。（图18）

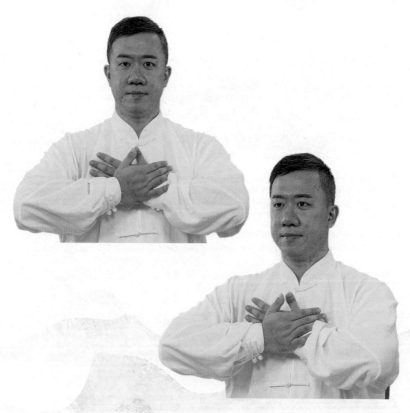

图18　左手小鱼际置于膻中穴按压、揉按（正侧位演示）

◎　调息操作要点：整个过程平静呼吸，在向下按压开始时呼气，放松时吸气，呼吸均匀舒缓。

　　◎　调心操作要点：心无旁骛，意守丹田，两目轻合，想象胸中滞气逐渐消散。

◎ 功法作用 ◎

　　膻中，属任脉，位于前正中线，平第4肋间，两乳头连线的中点，在胸骨体上；主治气喘、胸痛、心悸、心烦等。按揉膻中穴，可以缓解高血压和失眠患者的胸部憋闷、疼痛或心悸等症状。

调养功法

第七式
挦按肾俞身常暖

～ 调身操作要点：双手
成掌，按于腰背部足太阳膀胱
经肾俞穴位置，沿膀胱经循行
向下挦按至关元俞，每次挦按
均从上至下，共进行6次，以
感觉腰间微微发热为度。（图
19、图20）

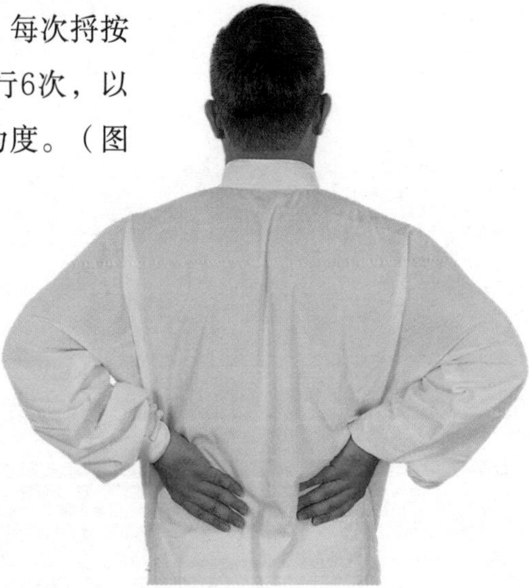

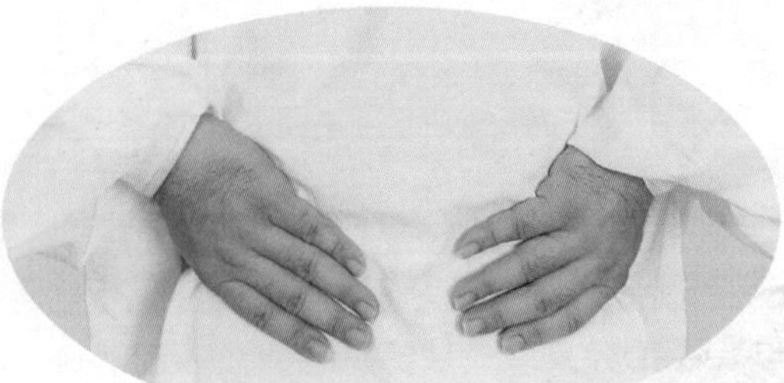

图19　双手成掌按于腰背部足太阳膀胱经肾俞穴
（及手部细节）

调息操作要点：向下捋按时缓缓呼气，恢复至原位过程中吸气，呼吸均匀舒缓。

调心操作要点：心无旁骛，意守丹田，两目轻合，想象腰间有暖流涌动。

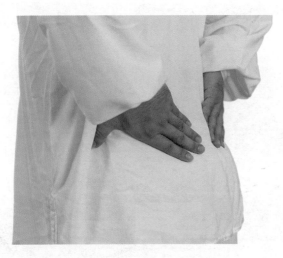

图20　沿膀胱经循行向下捋按至关元俞

肾俞，是足太阳膀胱经的常用腧穴之一，位于第2腰椎棘突下，旁开1.5寸，在腰背筋膜、最长肌和髂肋肌之间；主治腰痛、耳鸣、耳聋等。本功法自上而下，通过捋按肾俞穴调补肾气，填精补脑。

调养功法

☯ 第八式
点压脾肾脑髓充

　　☁ **调身操作要点：** 双手自大腿向下捋按至血海穴，用拇指点压血海穴6次；至足三里穴，用拇指点压足三里穴6次；至三阴交穴，用拇指点压三阴交穴6次。如此循环4遍。（图21～图23）

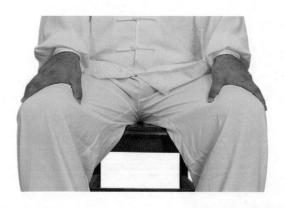

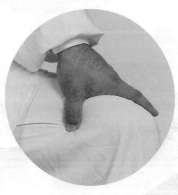

图21　双手自大腿向下
捋按至血海穴并点压

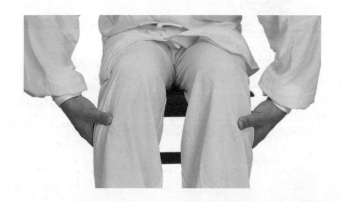

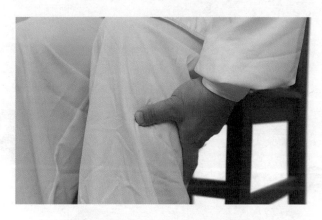

图22 捋按至足三里穴并点压（正侧位演示）

  调息操作要点：向下捋按时缓缓呼气，恢复至原位过程中吸气，呼吸均匀舒缓。

  调心操作要点：心无旁骛，意守丹田，两目轻合，想象大腿有暖流向下流动。

常见心血管病调养功法

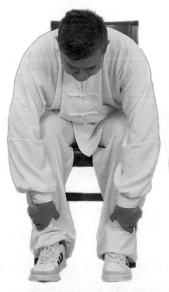

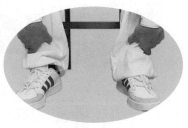

图23　捋按至三阴交穴并点压
（及局部细节）

❧ 功法作用 ❧

　　足三里，是足阳明胃经的主要穴位之一，在小腿外侧，犊鼻下3寸，犊鼻与解溪连线上；主治胃肠病症、下肢痿痹、神志病、外科疾患、虚劳诸证。三阴交，为足太阴脾经常用腧穴之一，为足三阴经（肝、脾、肾）的交会穴，在小腿内侧，当足内踝尖上3寸，胫骨内侧缘后方；常按压此穴可调补肝、脾、肾三经气血，对治疗内分泌失调，防治高血压、糖尿病、冠心病等效果显著。血海，屈膝在大腿内侧，髌底内侧端上2寸，当股四头肌内侧头的隆起处；血海是生血和活血化瘀的要穴。全方位按揉这三个穴位，可以调节肝肾、行气活血、改善症状。

第九式
点按太冲气自安

〰️ 调身操作要点：左腿横搭在右侧大腿上，右手拇指点压太冲穴6次，以感受到酸痛为度；左手拇指点按涌泉穴，共6次，以酸胀为度。左右脚交替，共进行4遍。（图24、图25）

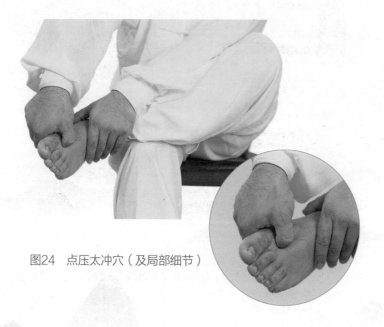

图24　点压太冲穴（及局部细节）

〰️ 调息操作要点：向下点按时呼气，动作稍缓，恢复至原位过程中吸气，呼吸均匀舒缓。

〰️ 调心操作要点：心无旁骛，意守丹田。

调养功法

常见心血管病调养功法

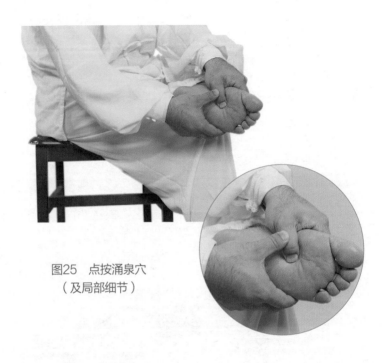

图25　点按涌泉穴
（及局部细节）

༄ 功法作用 ༄

　　太冲，属足厥阴肝经，位于足背，在第1、第2跖
骨间，跖骨底结合部前方凹陷处；具有疏肝理气、清
泻肝胆、清热泻火、平肝潜阳、疏经通络的功效。点
压太冲穴，可以起到缓解头痛、头晕症状，疏肝解郁
的功效。

☯ 收势

　　静坐闭目，含胸收腹，双腿自然落地，双手放于腿上，平稳呼吸，可吞咽口中津液，3分钟后缓缓站起，功法结束。

扫码即可观看
降压助眠功法

心功能不全调治 ⌇
——补气强身功法

　　该功法以改善心力衰竭患者或体质虚弱者的身体状况
为目的，根据中医学、针灸学、推拿学相关理论，结合彭
博士多年的养生功法训练及研究创立。该功法以点、按、
揉、压等按摩手法为基础，通过局部穴位的刺激及小范围
的身体运动调节气血的运行，达到补气温阳、养阴活血利
水的目的，从而治疗心力衰竭、虚劳、疲劳综合征等相关
疾病。

　　该功法将人体的作用位置分为了三大部分，分别是：
头颈部、上肢躯干、下肢足部。以上肢躯干动作为主，辅
以头颈部、下肢足部按摩增强疗效。头颈部主要干预穴
位为：百会、印堂。上肢躯干主要干预穴位为：内关、膻
中、关元、中极、气海。下肢足部主要干预穴位为：足三
里、三阴交、涌泉。

功法顺序：从上到下，由左及右。

☯ 起势

采取卧位、靠坐式均可。以靠坐式为例。

～ 调身操作要点：全身放松，靠坐椅上，两目轻闭，舌抵上颚，两唇微闭，脊背挺直，双手自然下垂，两足微分，与肩同宽。（图26）

～ 调息操作要点：自然呼吸，心情平静，腹式呼吸。

～ 调心操作要点：精神放松，意守丹田。

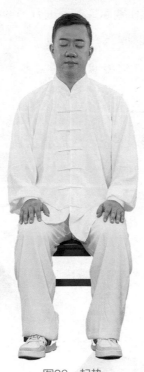

图26　起势

☯ 第一式
静心抵颚益气阴

⌒ **调身操作要点**：舌抵上颚，用适度力量抵压，每进行6次抵压，休息5秒之后，继续进行6次抵压；共进行4遍，然后将口内所生津液缓缓咽下。（图27）

⌒ **调息操作要点**：在抵压过程中，抵压时呼气，放松时吸气；抵压过程中平静呼吸，速度不宜过快，呼吸一次，抵压一次。

⌒ **调心操作要点**：心无旁骛，意守丹田。

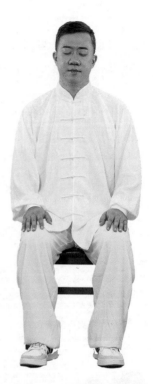

图27　舌抵上颚，用适度力量抵压

⌒ 功法作用 ⌒

在第一式中通过舌抵上颚生成的口中津液，中医认为具有滋阴补肾之功效，实践证明可以缓解患者口干、口苦症状。

☯ 第二式
点压印堂头目明

⌒ **调身操作要点:** 双手呈"八"字状,双手食指点压印堂穴,共点压6次,然后左手食指逆时针、右手食指顺时针揉按印堂穴6次;共重复4遍。(图28)

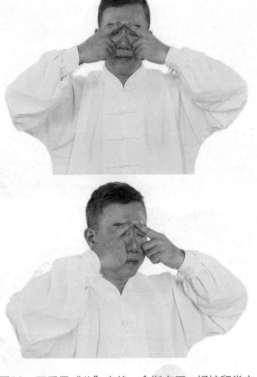

图28 双手呈"八"字状,食指点压、揉按印堂穴
(正侧位演示)

ᴄ 调息操作要点：整个过程平静呼吸，点压印堂穴时呼气，放松时吸气。

ᴄ 调心操作要点：心无旁骛，意守丹田，想象一团气聚集于印堂部位。

ᴄ 功法作用 ᴄ

印堂，属于经外奇穴。此腧穴位于人体额部，在两眉头的中间。有明目通鼻、宁心安神的作用，临床上主要用于配合治疗失眠、头痛等症状。点压印堂穴，可以改善心功能不全患者睡眠，缓解患者头痛等症状。

第三式
按揉任脉阳气升

✐ 调身操作要点：双手成掌，按于腹部任脉关元穴、气海穴位置，轻微用力，以感觉手心发热为度，共按压6次；然后逆时针揉按关元穴、气海穴位置，共进行6次，以感觉下腹部微微发热为度；共重复4遍。（图29）

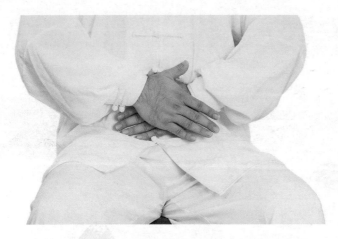

图29　按压及揉按关元穴、气海穴

   调息操作要点：按压及揉按过程中缓缓呼气，恢复至原位过程中吸气，呼吸均匀舒缓。

   调心操作要点：心无旁骛，意守丹田，两目轻合，想象下腹部丹田部位有暖流涌动。

功法作用

关元，属任脉，足三阴、任脉之会，小肠募穴。在下腹部，前正中线上，当脐中下3寸。主治中风脱证、肾虚气喘、遗精、阳痿、疝气、遗尿、淋浊、尿频、尿闭、子宫脱垂、神经衰弱、晕厥、休克等，并有强壮作用。气海，属任脉，肓之原穴。在下腹部，前正中线上，当脐中下1.5寸。主治虚脱、厥逆、腹痛、泄泻、月经不调、痛经、崩漏、带下、遗精、阳痿、遗尿、疝气及尿潴留、尿路感染、肠梗阻等，具有强壮作用。关元和气海作为中医经典的具有补益气血、温补阳气作用的穴位，使用按揉或者艾灸等方法均具有较好的临床疗效，可以改善心功能不全患者虚弱、乏力、性功能下降等诸多虚弱症状。

☯ 第四式

点压三里脾胃健

～ **调身操作要点：** 双手拇指点压足三里穴6次，然后左手拇指逆时针、右手拇指顺时针揉按足三里穴6次；共重复4遍。（图30）

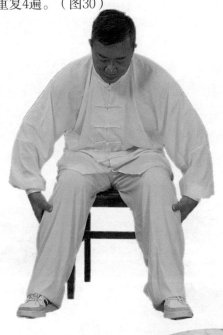

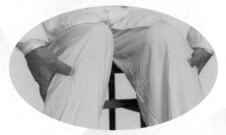

图30　点压、揉按足三里穴（及局部细节）

    ◎ 调息操作要点：向下按压时缓缓呼气，恢复至原位过程中吸气，呼吸均匀舒缓。

    ◎ 调心操作要点：心无旁骛，意守丹田，两目轻合，想象有暖流聚集于足三里部位。

功法作用

    足三里，是足阳明胃经的主要穴位之一，在小腿外侧，犊鼻下3寸，犊鼻与解溪连线上；主治胃肠病症、下肢痿痹、神志病、外科疾患、虚劳诸证。足三里作为中医学经典的强壮要穴，具有补脾益气、强壮补虚的作用，长期坚持揉按，对于改善心功能不全患者的虚弱症状具有良好疗效。

☯ 第五式
点揉三阴津液盈

    ⌒ 调身操作要点：右腿横搭在左侧大腿上，双手拇指点压三阴交穴6次，然后左手拇指逆时针、右手拇指顺时针揉按三阴交穴6次。左右脚交替，共进行4遍。（图31）

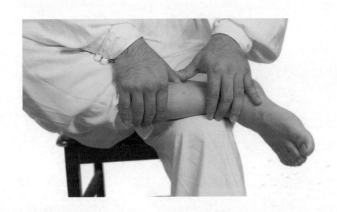

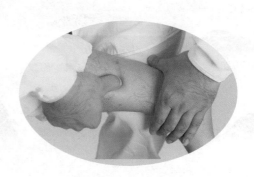

图31　点压、揉按三阴交穴（及局部细节）

  调息操作要点：向下按压时缓缓呼气，恢复至原位过程中吸气，呼吸均匀舒缓。

  调心操作要点：心无旁骛，意守丹田，两目轻合，想象有暖流聚集于三阴交部位。

❧ 功法作用 ❧

  三阴交，为足太阴脾经常用腧穴之一，为足三阴经（肝、脾、肾）的交会穴，在小腿内侧，当足内踝尖上3寸，胫骨内侧缘后方。常按压此穴可调补肝、脾、肾三经气血，长期坚持揉按，对于改善心功能不全患者的肝肾阴虚症状具有良好疗效。

第六式
揉按涌泉气顺宁

↩ 调身操作要点：右腿横搭在左侧大腿上，右手拇指点按涌泉穴共6次，以酸胀为度，然后拇指揉按涌泉穴6次；左右脚交替，共进行4遍。（图32）

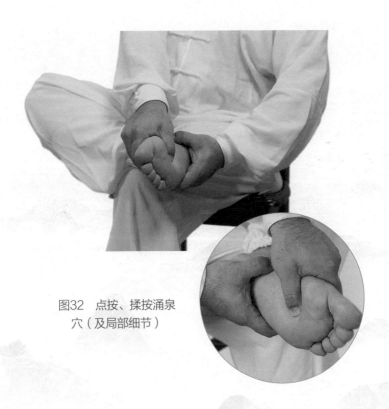

图32　点按、揉按涌泉
　　　穴（及局部细节）

调养功法

039

　　☙ 调息操作要点：向下点按时呼气，动作稍缓，恢复至原位过程中吸气，呼吸均匀舒缓。

　　☙ 调心操作要点：心无旁骛，意守丹田，想象气聚于涌泉穴位置。

☙ 功法作用 ☙

　　涌泉，是足少阴肾经的常用腧穴之一，位于足底部，蜷足时足前部凹陷处，约当足底第2、第3跖趾缝纹头端与足跟连线的前1/3与后2/3交点上。主治肺系病症、大便难、小便不利、奔豚气。揉按涌泉穴可以通利二便、滋阴补肾，对于改善心功能不全患者腑气不通及肝肾阴虚症状有较好疗效。

☯ 收势

　　静坐闭目，含胸收腹，双腿自然分开，双手放于体侧，平稳呼吸，可吞咽口中津液，5分钟后缓缓坐起，功法结束。

扫码即可观看
补气强身功法

调养功法

眩晕调治 ～
——整脊松项功法

    该功法以改善颈椎病、肩周炎和颈肩腰腿痛患者的身体状况为目的，根据中医学、针灸学、推拿学相关理论，结合彭博士多年的养生功法训练及研究创立。该功法以局部关节转动及全身运动为主，通过指导患者进行自身相应的运动调节气血的运行，达到舒筋活血，松调关节的目的，从而治疗颈椎病、肩周炎及颈肩腰腿痛等。

    该功法将人体的作用位置分为了三大部分，分别是：头颈部、上肢躯干、下肢足部。以头颈部动作为主，辅以上肢躯干、下肢足部动作增强疗效。

功法顺序：从上到下，由左及右。

☯ 起势

采取立位、坐位均可。以立位为例。

⌒ 调身操作要点：全身放松，自然站立，两目轻闭，舌抵上颚，两唇微闭，松肩垂肘，手放体侧；两足微分，与肩同宽。（图33）

⌒ 调息操作要点：自然呼吸，心情平静，腹式呼吸。

⌒ 调心操作要点：精神放松，意守丹田。

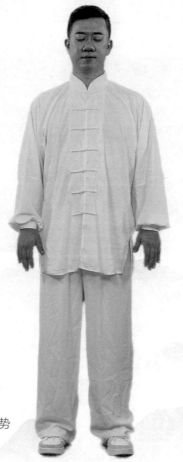

图33　起势

常见心血管病调养功法

☯ 第一式
仰面转头颈项舒

〰 调身操作要点：头仰向后，面朝上，然后复位，如此循环6次；头保持中正，平转向左侧，复位，如此循环4次；头保持中正，平转向右侧，复位，如此循环4次。（图34）

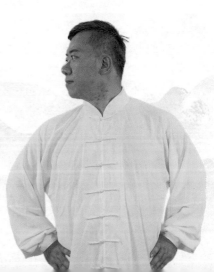

图34　头保持中正平，转向左/右侧（及整体演示）

ン 调息操作要点：自然呼吸，心情平静，腹式呼吸。

ン 调心操作要点：精神放松，意守丹田，呼吸均匀。

ン 功法作用 ン

　　头部左右旋转、上下抬举，可以增强颈部深浅肌
群的收缩能力，同时头颈部运动对于调节脏腑气血和协
调全身均有作用。锻炼颈部肌群，有助于治疗落枕和颈
椎病，减轻眩晕和上肢麻木，改善颈部酸痛等症状。

调养功法

📿 第二式
转肩松肩关节灵

　　☁ 调身操作要点：双肩向前画圈6次，暂停3秒，双肩向后画圈6次，暂停3秒。如此循环4遍。（图35）

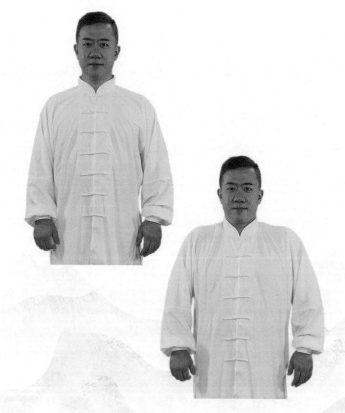

图35　双肩向前/后画圈

- 调息操作要点: 自然呼吸，心情平静，腹式呼吸。
- 调心操作要点: 精神放松，意守丹田，呼吸均匀。

☙ 功法作用 ❧

　　转肩，可以增强肩关节活动度，改善肩部灵活性，改善局部血液循环，对于缓解肩周炎和肩部酸痛不适具有良好作用。

🌓 第三式

俯仰怀抱脊康健

～ 调身操作要点：两臂上举过头，向后轻度过伸，维持3秒；向前俯身，两手尽量触地，维持3秒；身体下蹲，双手抱肩，维持3秒。如此循环4遍。（图36～图38）

～ 调息操作要点：自然呼吸，心情平静，腹式呼吸。

～ 调心操作要点：精神放松，呼吸均匀。

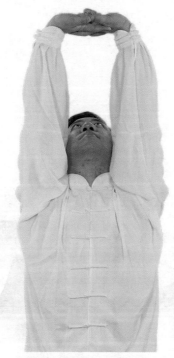

图36　两臂上举过头，
向后轻度过伸

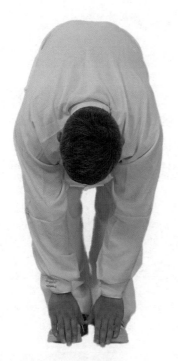 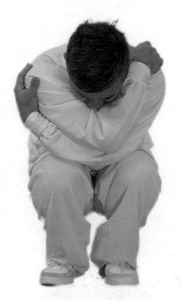

图37　向前俯身，
　　　两手尽量触地

图38　身体下蹲，
　　　双手抱肩

❧ 功法作用 ❧

　　这一段动作，包括头向后仰，上体背伸、前屈和弯腰，主要运动脊柱。脊柱是全身运动的中枢，又是头颈和躯干负重的轴心。脊柱运动不仅能加强颈部、胸部、腰部肌肉，以及颈椎、胸椎、腰椎关节及韧带等连结的活动能力，而且对于支配下肢的主要神经（如坐骨神经），有良好的调节作用。

调养功法

常见心血管病调养功法

☯ 第四式
旋转动摇腰转灵

🌀 调身操作要点：双手叉腰，腰部先逆时针旋转4周，休息3秒；然后顺时针旋转4周，休息3秒。如此循环3遍。（图39）

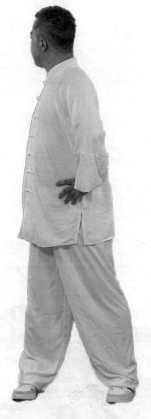
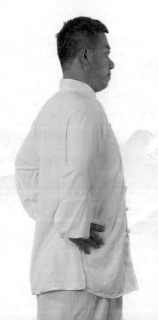

图39　双手叉腰，旋转腰部

◌ 调息操作要点：自然呼吸，心情平静，腹式呼吸。

◌ 调心操作要点：精神放松，呼吸均匀。

◌ **功法作用** ◌

　　本段动作主要活动腰部肌肉、关节，通过旋转腰部，促进局部肌肉韧带活动，起到行气活血化瘀的功效，可以改善患者腰部酸痛、乏力的症状。

调养功法

☯ 收势

　　闭目，含胸收腹，双腿自然分开，双手放于体侧，平稳呼吸，可吞咽口中津液，5分钟后功法结束。

扫码即可观看
整脊松项功法

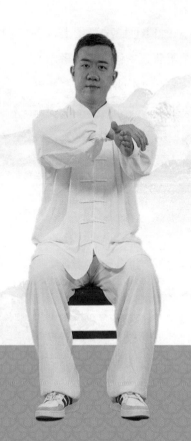

常见心血管病调养功法

常见心血管病
相关科普知识

高血压 ～

什么是高血压?

在未使用降压药物的情况下，非同日3次测量上肢血压，收缩压≥140 mmHg和（或）舒张压≥90 mmHg考虑为高血压。目前90%以上的高血压原因尚不明确，为"原发性高血压"。如果血压高是由某些疾病（如肾脏病、原发性醛固酮增多症、嗜铬细胞瘤等）引起的，为"继发性高血压"。继发性高血压服药治疗的效果差，当针对病因治疗，去除病因后血压能有效降低甚至恢复正常。

什么人易得高血压?

高血压的易患对象有：摄盐过多，进食高热量食物而缺乏活动所致的超重、肥胖，长期过量饮酒、吸烟、缺乏运动，长期精神压力大，有高血压家族史，55岁及以上的男性和更年期后的女性。有以上危险因素之一者，建议每6个月测量一次血压，改变不良生活方式，防止高血压的发生。

高血压有什么可怕？

大多数高血压患者通常无症状，许多患者根本不知道自己血压高，在体检或偶尔测血压时才发现血压高，故高血压被称为"无声杀手"。有些患者是在发生了心脏病、脑卒中、肾功能衰竭时才知道自己的血压高。所以，建议血压正常的成人每两年至少测量一次血压。各级医疗机构应强化首诊测血压制度，患者就诊，不管看什么病，都要测量血压，以便早发现高血压、早治疗。有头晕、头痛、眼花、耳鸣、失眠、心悸、气促、胸闷、肥胖、打鼾、乏力、记忆力减退、肢体无力或麻痹、夜尿增多、泡沫尿等症状，表明可能血压高，应尽快就诊。

持续的血压升高可造成心、脑、肾、全身血管及眼部的损害，严重时可发生脑卒中、心肌梗死、心力衰竭、肾功能衰竭、主动脉夹层等危及生命的临床并发症。

心脏：高血压可引起左心室肥厚、冠心病、心力衰竭和心律失常。①左心室肥厚：左心室肥厚是高血压最常见的靶器官损害。血压升高使心脏向动脉射血的阻力增大、负担加重，心腔内压力高，加上一些神经体液因子的作用，造成心肌细胞肥大、间质纤维化，导致心肌肥厚。②冠心病：高血压促进动脉粥样硬化的进展。随着血压水平的升高，冠心病发病概率也随之增高。高血压患者发生冠心病的概率较血压正常者高2.6倍。③心力衰竭：心肌肥厚及动脉粥样硬化造成心肌供血不足，心脏舒张和

常见心血管病相关科普知识

收缩功能受损，最终发生心力衰竭。患者会出现夜间呼吸困难，劳累或饱食时发生气喘、心悸、咳嗽，少尿、水肿等症状。④心律失常：由于心肌肥厚、缺血和纤维化，心室肥厚患者容易发生室性心律失常，甚至猝死。心房颤动是高血压患者常见的一种心律失常，心房颤动易在左心房形成血栓，血栓可脱落，阻塞血管，如果阻塞脑动脉则会引起脑卒中。

脑：我国是脑卒中高发区，年新发脑卒中患者250万人。高血压是脑卒中最重要的危险因素，我国70%的脑卒中患者患有高血压。高血压可引起脑梗死、脑出血、短暂性脑缺血发作等。①脑梗死：原因有二，其一，颅内动脉硬化，原位血栓形成；其二，颅外的栓子（例如颈动脉粥样斑块脱落、心房颤动患者左心房血栓脱落），随血流堵塞脑部动脉。②腔隙性脑梗死：长期高血压使脑小动脉硬化，血管腔狭窄闭塞，缺血区脑组织坏死软化，形成2～15 mm的病灶，残留小囊腔，为腔隙性脑梗死；反复发作出现多个囊腔者，为多发性腔隙性脑梗死，会造成脑萎缩以至于老年性痴呆。③脑出血：脑内小动脉硬化变脆，在高压力下膨出形成动脉瘤，甚者破裂，引起脑出血；脑出血的病情凶险。④短暂性脑缺血发作：俗称"小中风"，为脑卒中的先兆。表现为肢体短暂性的活动障碍、麻木无力，或眩晕、黑矇、失语、吞咽困难，持续数十分钟，24 h内完全恢复，不遗留症状，可反复发作，每次发作表现基本相同。1/3的患者将在5年内发展成脑梗死，发生心肌梗死的可能性也很高。

肾脏：长期高血压使肾小球内压力增高，造成肾小球损害和肾微小动脉病变，一般在高血压持续10～15年后出现肾损害、肾功能减退，部分患者可发展成肾功能衰竭。

血管：高血压患者大多伴有动脉粥样硬化，下肢动脉因粥样硬化发生狭窄或闭塞时，出现间歇性跛行，重者可有下肢静息痛甚至溃疡或坏疽。主动脉夹层是指主动脉内膜撕裂，血流把主动脉壁的内膜和中层剥离，形成壁内血肿。典型者可表现为突发的胸腹部撕裂样剧痛，病情非常凶险，可伴休克，甚至猝死。如有间断的胸痛、腹痛伴发热等症状，需注意不典型主动脉夹层的可能。

眼：高血压可损害眼底动脉、视网膜、视神经，造成眼底视网膜小动脉硬化、视网膜出血和渗出、视网膜中央动脉或静脉阻塞、视乳头水肿萎缩、黄斑变性等，致视力下降，重者失明。

得了高血压该怎么吃？

每天摄入少量（2～3 g）食盐是人体维持生命的必需，但过量食盐摄入（＞6 g/d）会导致不良生理反应，其中最主要的就是血压升高。研究证明，盐的摄入量与血压水平呈正相关，严格控制钠盐摄入可有效控制血压。钾能促钠排出，钾的摄入量与血压水平呈负相关，我国居民的膳食特点是低钾高钠。我国人群每天钾的摄入量只有1.89 g，远低于世界卫生组织（WHO）建议的4.7 g。

我国南方人群钠盐摄入量平均为8～10 g/d，北方人群为12～15 g/d，均远远超过WHO建议的5 g的标准。高盐膳食不仅是高血压发生的主要危险因素，也是脑卒中、心脏病和肾脏病发生发展的危险因素。每日摄入的钠盐从9 g降至6 g，可使脑卒中发病率下降22%，冠心病发病率下降16%。

得了高血压该怎么运动？

我国城市居民（尤其是中青年）普遍缺乏体力活动，严重影响心血管健康。体力活动不足是高血压的危险因素。适量运动可缓解交感神经紧张，增加扩血管物质，改善内皮舒张功能，促进糖脂代谢，降低血压，降低心血管疾病患病风险。运动中的收缩压随运动强度增加而升高，中等强度运动时收缩压可比安静状态升高30～50 mmHg，舒张压有轻微变化或基本维持稳定。运动可降低安静时的血压，每次10 min以上中低强度运动的降压效果可以维持10～22 h，长期坚持规律运动，可以增强运动带来的降压效果。安静时血压超过180/110 mmHg的患者，暂时禁止中度及以上的运动。高血压患者适宜的运动方式有：有氧运动、力量练习、柔韧性练习、综合功能练习。

有氧运动：有氧运动是高血压患者最基本的健身方式，常见运动形式有快走、慢跑、骑自行车、秧歌舞、广播体操、有氧健身操、登山、爬楼梯等。建议每周至少进行3～5次、每次30 min以上中等强度的有氧运动,最好坚持每天都运动。在降血压方面中、低强度运动较高强度运动更有效、更安全。可选用以下方法评估中等运动强度:①主观感觉:运动中心跳加快、微微出汗、自我感觉有点累。②客观表现:运动中呼吸频率加快、微微喘,可以与人交谈,但是不能唱歌。③步行速度:每分钟120步左右。④运动中的心率≈170-年龄。⑤在休息约10 min内,锻炼所引起的呼吸频率增加应明显缓解,心率也恢复到正常或接近正常。

力量练习:力量练习可以增加肌肉量,增强肌肉力量,减缓关节疼痛,增强人体平衡能力,防止跌倒,改善血压。建议高血压患者每周进行2～3次力量练习,每次练习间隔48 h以上。可采用多种运动方式和器械设备,对每一个主要肌群进行力量练习,每组力量练习以重复10～15次为宜。生活中的推、拉、拽、举、压等动作都是力量练习的方式。力量练习应选择中低强度,练习时应保持正常呼吸状态,避免憋气。

柔韧性练习:柔韧性练习可以改善关节活动度,增强人体的协调性和平衡能力,防止摔倒。建议每周进行2～3次柔韧性练习。练习时,每次拉伸达到拉紧或轻微不适状态时应保持10～30 s,每一个部位的拉伸可以重复2～4次,共计60 s。

综合功能练习:综合功能练习可以增强人体的灵敏度和协调性,改善步态、身体功能,防止跌倒,包括太极、瑜伽、太极柔力球、乒乓球、羽毛球等。

　　另外，生活中适当增加体力活动有助于控制血压。高血压患者可以适当做些家务、步行购物等，每天的步行总数达到或接近10 000步为宜。高血压患者的血压在清晨常处于比较高的水平，清晨也是心血管事件的高发时段，因此最好选择下午或傍晚进行锻炼。

🌑 得了高血压该怎么治疗？

　　"降压是硬道理"：早降压早获益；长期降压长期获益；降压达标，将高血压患者的心血管风险降到最低，最大获益。

　　降压药的用药原则：小剂量开始；优先应用长效制剂；联合用药；个体化。

　　血压控制的目标：一般高血压<140/90 mmHg；老年高血压<150/90 mmHg。

　　血压达标时间：一般患者用药后4～12周内达标，高龄、冠状动脉或双颈动脉严重狭窄及耐受性差的患者达标时间适当延长。

　　常用降压药有钙通道阻滞药（CCB）、血管紧张素转化酶抑制剂（ACEI）、血管紧张素受体阻滞药（ARB）、利尿剂、β受体阻滞剂及单片复方制剂（SPC），均可用于高血压初始和维持治疗，各有其特点和适应证。

　　高血压患者应长期治疗和定期随访。

中医是怎么认识高血压的?

"高血压",是现代医学病名。中医学中,没有"高血压"的病名和作为专病的记载,在古籍中则多分散记录,属于中医认识内"头痛""眩晕"范畴。若病情进一步发展,出现器官损害时,还有可能出现"心悸""怔忡""胸痹""水肿""中风"等症状。

《医学衷中参西录》中将高血压称为"脑充血病"。1997年,国家技术监督局制定《中医临床诊疗术语·疾病部分》对常见中医病名进行了规范,将高血压的中医病名定为"风眩",释义为"风眩是以眩晕、头痛、血压增高、脉弦等为主要表现的眩晕类疾病"。

高血压的发生,主要是由于七情六欲不节、饮食劳伤或年老体虚导致的风、痰、火等病理产物影响肝、肾、心、脾等脏腑功能。更年期前后女性患病率迅速升高,与冲任二脉的经气盛衰变化密切相关。证型有虚证、实证,也有虚实夹杂证,故应当慎重地辨证施治。治法主要有平肝、镇痉、理血、补益等。

高血压的中医治疗方案

在中医领域里,高血压病的主要辨证分型及治疗方案有以下几种。

痰浊内蕴型:症见头晕头痛、头重、呕恶胸闷、舌质暗红、舌苔黄腻或白腻、脉滑等;治疗以健脾祛湿、化痰息风为主；传统方药有半夏白术天麻汤、泽泻汤等。

肝阳上亢型：症见头晕头痛、耳鸣耳聋、失眠、腰膝酸软、烦热易怒、心悸、舌红苔黄或少苔，脉弦、数、细等；治疗以平肝潜阳、补益肝肾、清热祛火为主；传统方药有天麻钩藤饮、镇肝息风汤、建瓴汤等。

肝肾阴虚型：症见头晕、耳鸣耳聋、腰膝酸软、失眠、五心烦热、舌红少苔，脉弦细数等；治疗以补肾滋肝、安神养心为主；传统方药有杞菊地黄汤等。

冲任失调型：症见阴虚阳亢，除头晕、烘热汗出、五心烦热外，还应有冲任失调、月经不规律等，与女性围绝经期的特殊生理时期有明显的关系；治疗以调理冲任、清泻虚火为主；传统方药有二仙汤等。

瘀血阻络型：症见麻木、头晕头痛、胸痛、刺痛、痛有定处，舌紫暗有瘀斑、舌下络脉异常，脉弦涩等；治疗以活血化瘀为主，多采用活血化瘀方加减；传统方药有通窍活血汤等。

阴阳两虚型：症见头晕怕冷、耳鸣耳聋、腰膝酸软、疲乏、少气心悸、小便频数、舌淡苔白，脉沉、细等；治疗以滋阴助阳为主；传统方药有八珍汤或十全大补汤等。

高血压的临床治疗主要采用药物治疗方法，并配合以生活管理，有效降低血压的同时，减少血压异常升高的诱发因素。但是高血压无法根治，因此需要在长期、持续的治疗和护理当中，维持血压的稳定，控制病情的进展。在高血压治疗中，中医药方法是一种良好的治疗选择。此外，还可配合针灸等中医特色疗法。

🍃 高血压的食疗

《饮食辨录》中云："饮食得宜足为药饵之助，失宜则反与药饵为仇"。食疗是医疗和膳食之间连接最为密切的桥梁。高血压作为一种常见病和多发病，常伴有肥胖、高血脂及糖尿病等，这些疾病都与饮食息息相关。因此，通过中医食疗对日常饮食进行干预，从而预防或辅助治疗高血压，是势在必行的。

针对高血压，推荐部分食疗方案如下。

肝阳上亢型高血压患者：宜以偏凉性食物为佳，如萝卜、芹菜和紫菜等；少吃辛辣及易上火食物，如辣椒、葱、蒜等。食疗方有玉米须炖猪蹄、山楂降压汤等。

痰浊内蕴型高血压患者：宜素食，以祛痰、健脾食物为主，如芹菜、山楂、山药等。食疗方有洋葱炒肉片、橘皮饮等。

阴阳两虚型高血压患者：宜同时补阴补阳，补阴类食物有梨、葡萄、荸荠、甘蔗、黄瓜等。补阳类食物有核桃仁、荔枝干、黑枣、桂圆等。食疗方有枸杞桂圆羊肉汤和鸡肝熟地黄汤等。

气血亏虚型高血压患者：以滋补食物为主，如瘦肉、鱼、蛋、红枣、党参等补益气血食物。食疗方有黄芪大枣粥、归参炖母鸡等。

整体上，食疗方案以清淡饮食为指导，坚持低盐、低脂、低糖和低胆固醇饮食，同时根据自身的体质情况进行相应的禁食调整，尤其应戒烟酒。还需要多吃水果、蔬菜，适当补充钙、钾及相关的维生素，促进胆固醇排出，同时保护自身的心血管功能。

🌰 高血压病的发展简史及《中国高血压防治指南》20年变迁

∽ 什么是血压?

血压是指血液在血管内流动时作用于单位面积血管壁的侧压力，检查所测量的一般是体循环的动脉血压，包括收缩压和舒张压。

∽ 血压计的发明

1733年英国皇家学会斯蒂芬·黑尔斯（Stephen Hales，1677—1761）首次测量了动物的血压。他用尾端接有小金属管的长9英尺（274 cm）直径1/6英寸（4.23 mm）的玻璃管插入一匹马的颈动脉，此时血液立即涌入玻璃管内，高达8.3英尺（270 cm），并维持270 cm的柱高。

俄国外科医生尼古拉·柯洛特科夫（Nikolai Korotkoff，1874—1920）在测血压时，加上了听诊器。这一点改进使血压测量飞跃到一个全新的水平，直到现在仍然是血压测量的基本方法。从此，人们对高血压的认识进入快车道。

∽ 高血压病及《中国高血压防治指南》的发展

1957年，Framingham研究首次定义高血压为血压≥160/95 mmHg，把高血压带进了数值时代，高血压正式成为一种疾病。

1999年首部《中国高血压防治指南》（以下简称《指南》）发布，首次提出了140/90 mmHg的高血压诊断标准，中国的高血压防治进入"140/90 mmHg"时代。

高血压各类人群的降压目标

1999年至2018年的四版《指南》针对一般高血压患者的降压目标值在不断更新，针对高血压特殊人群的目标血压值更为细化。1999年版《指南》建议青年人、中年人或糖尿病患者降压至理想或正常血压＜130/85 mmHg；2005年版和2010年版《指南》均建议普通高血压患者的降压目标值控制在140/90 mmHg以下。但2005年版《指南》首次提出老年患者的血压应降至＜150/90 mmHg，这也是区别于国际上其他指南的一点。

2018年版《指南》对于高血压患者的血压控制趋于严格，提出了"双目标"的要求：①对于一般高血压患者应降至＜140/90 mmHg；能耐受者和部分高危及以上的患者可进一步降至＜130/80 mmHg。②对于65～79岁的老年患者首先应降至＜150/90 mmHg；如能耐受，可进一步降至＜140/90 mmHg。③80岁及以上的老年患者应降至＜150/90 mmHg。

高血压药物治疗原则

1999年至2018年，《中国高血压防治指南》对降压药物的推荐种类显著增加，肾素-血管紧张素系统抑制剂

（RASI）的适应证和治疗地位显著提升，对β受体阻滞剂的推荐无明显变化。四版《指南》中药物治疗原则的变化大致有以下三点：①药物剂量的变化，采用小剂量到逐渐增加至足剂量。②长效药物推荐力度逐渐加大。③起始联合治疗的门槛降低。

《中国高血压防治指南》越来越重视联合治疗，2018年版《指南》特别强调单片复方制剂（SPC）是联合治疗的新趋势。与随机组方的降压联合治疗相比，SPC联合治疗的优点是使用方便，可改善治疗的依从性及疗效。尤其是基于ACEI/ARB的联合治疗（表1），优先推荐使用SPC。

表1　以RAS抑制剂为基础的联合治疗方案推荐

主要推荐应用的优化联合治疗方案	可以考虑使用的联合治疗方案	不常规推荐但必要时可慎用的联合治疗方案
二氢吡啶类CCB+ARB	利尿剂+β受体阻滞剂	ACEI+β受体阻滞剂
二氢吡啶类CCB+ACEI	α受体阻滞剂+β受体阻滞剂	ARB+β受体阻滞剂
ARB+噻嗪类利尿剂	二氢吡啶类CCB+保钾利尿剂	ACEI+ARB
ACEI+噻嗪类利尿剂	噻嗪类利尿剂+保钾利尿剂	中枢作用药+β受体阻滞剂
二氢吡啶类CCB+噻嗪类利尿剂	—	—
二氢吡啶类CCB+β受体阻滞剂	—	—

心功能不全 ⌒
——心力衰竭

● 什么是心力衰竭?

心力衰竭是指心功能发生改变,心脏收缩力下降使心排血量不能满足机体代谢的需要,器官、组织血液供应不足,同时出现肺循环和(或)体循环瘀血而表现出的一系列症状。

根据发病的部位可分为左心衰、右心衰和全心衰。左心衰时肺静脉回流受阻,会导致肺水肿,临床多见咳嗽、咳白色或粉红色浆液性泡沫痰、气喘,不能平卧;右心衰时腔静脉回流受阻,临床多见水肿(以下肢较明显)、尿少、肝充血肿大、颈静脉怒张。

根据发病的速度可分为急性心力衰竭和慢性心力衰竭。急性心力衰竭是正常或原有病损的心脏,由于心室负荷过重或其他因素,急骤发生明显的心肌收缩力减弱、心排血量减少,不足以适应身体需要,迅速引起静脉瘀血、水肿的临床综合征,可由感染、心律失常、体力活动或情绪紧张、妊娠或分娩、输血和输液、钠盐摄入过多以及对心肌有抑制作用的药物应用不当等引发。慢性心力衰竭，是指由各种慢性心血管病变引起的心力衰竭。

总而言之，心力衰竭并非一个独立的疾病，而是心脏疾病发展的终末阶段，是因心脏结构或功能异常导致心室充盈或射血功能发生障碍，从而出现的一系列症状和体征，主要表现为呼吸困难、乏力、水肿等。在原有慢性心脏疾病基础上逐渐出现心力衰竭体征的为慢性心衰；急性心衰可由慢性心衰演变而来，或见于急性心肌梗死和严重心肌炎。

心功能不全的程度，常使用纽约心功能分级（NYHA心功能分级）以评估。Ⅰ级：日常活动无心力衰竭症状。Ⅱ级：日常活动出现心力衰竭症状。Ⅲ级：低于日常活动出现心力衰竭症状。Ⅳ级：在休息时出现心力衰竭症状。

为什么会得心力衰竭？

心力衰竭的根本原因在于心脏泵血能力下降，因此有高血压、冠心病、糖尿病、心肌炎等影响心脏功能的心血管疾病的患者都属于心力衰竭的易患对象，可在积极治疗原有疾病的同时定期进行超声心动图和X线胸片检查。据我国部分地区42家医院，对10 714例心力衰竭住院病例的回顾性调查，其病因以冠心病居首，其次为高血压，因此重点关注防治高血压、冠心病对预防心力衰竭有重要作用。

心力衰竭有什么可怕?

心力衰竭最常见的症状包括呼吸困难、乏力、运动受限、血液瘀滞,其他症状包括夜尿增多、食欲减弱、腹胀与腹部不适、便秘及神经症状如意识模糊、头晕、记忆力障碍等。

心力衰竭是一种严重影响人身心健康的综合征,并常常伴有肺、肝脏、肾脏、血管等多器官脏器的损伤。

心脏:心力衰竭是一种进行性的病变,发病以后,即使没有新的心肌损害,临床表现稳定,病情仍然可以进一步加重。心力衰竭患者,由于心脏结构和功能的改变,可伴有室性心律失常并可能导致猝死;心力衰竭时,扩张的心室以及低下的收缩力,使得心室内血液瘀滞,容易发生血栓栓塞,引发心肌梗死或者脑梗死。

肺:左心衰肺静脉高压导致肺水肿,肺水肿早期表现为胸闷、气短、心悸、端坐呼吸,伴有轻度低氧血症;加重则表现为严重的呼吸困难、强迫端坐呼吸、紫绀、剧烈咳嗽、咳大量泡沫或粉红色泡沫痰,伴有严重低氧血症,并可能导致休克、呼吸衰竭、器官衰竭甚至死亡。

肝脏:体循环瘀滞,导致肝脏充血肿大,肝内瘀血形成心源性肝硬化、黄疸,肝细胞损伤会导致电解质紊乱。

肾脏:由于心收缩功能减退,排出血量减少,流经肾的血量减少,肌体的水盐排不出去就会形成水肿;此外体循环瘀血也会引起肾瘀血,肾功能损伤继而形成水肿。

血管：由于肾损伤，机体水排不出去，使得血容量增大，激活肾素-血管紧张素-醛固酮系统，使血压升高，高血压又会导致心肌肥厚，加重心力衰竭。

得了心力衰竭该怎么吃？

饮食以低热量、低钠、低脂、清淡易消化的食物为主，少食多餐。心力衰竭患者食欲和消化能力较差，饮食不应增加心脏、肠胃负担，同时应尽量补充优质蛋白质、维生素B族、维生素C等，保护心肌。

限制钠盐摄入。一般认为每日摄盐量以2～5 g为宜，晚期心力衰竭患者摄盐量每天以小于2 g为宜。临床试验显示，减少钠盐摄入量可以降低血压，而长期维持血压水平正常可以有效预防心血管病的发生。中国人钠盐摄入量普遍较高（平均10.5 g/d），如果钠盐摄入量不能立即降低至推荐水平，长期逐渐减少也可以有效降低发病风险。

限制水的摄入。水的多量摄入会使全身血液容量增多，心脏负担随之增加。轻度心力衰竭的患者，每日饮水量应控制在1 500 mL以内。

得了心力衰竭该怎么运动？

适度体力活动可以有效提高身体耐力，建议进行易于控制强度的有氧运动，如慢跑、打太极拳等。一次运动持续时间控制在半小时至一小时。慢性心力衰竭患者运动具有一定危险性，具体以医师开具的运动处方为准。

得了心力衰竭该怎么治疗?

慢性心力衰竭是各种心脏疾病的终末阶段,治疗时,原来各种基本病症,如高血压、冠心病、心肌炎、心包炎等,需要祛除或控制缓解,避免原病的复发与加重。

导致心力衰竭的机制是心室重构,预防或延缓心室重构可避免或减缓心力衰竭的发生。对此常用的药物有血管紧张素转化酶抑制剂(ACEI)、血管紧张素受体阻滞药(ARB)和盐皮质激素受体拮抗剂(MRA)、β受体阻滞剂和洋地黄制剂。

心力衰竭容易引起水肿,及时排出体内的水盐,可减轻心脏的负担。可用利尿剂减轻水肿,常用的有呋塞米(furosemide)、噻嗪类,如氯噻嗪(chlorothiazide)、氨苯蝶啶(triamterene)、阿米洛利(amiloride)。

心力衰竭是比较严重的心脏疾病,应密切观察病情变化并定期随访。

中医是怎么认识心力衰竭的?

中国古代并没有"心力衰竭"这一现代概念,但中医对心力衰竭的治疗却有悠久的历史。在中医认知中,心力衰竭引起的心率、心律异常是为心悸;心力衰竭引起肺水肿,使得呼吸不畅、气息急促是为喘促;心力衰竭使静脉回流受阻,引起肝充血、腹胀、腹水是为水饮;心力衰竭引起的下肢甚至周身水肿,是为水肿、阴肿;心力衰竭使静脉回流受阻而血液瘀滞，使面色、唇色色黯，舌下脉络迂曲是为瘀血。

中医认为心主血脉，心生血。《黄帝内经》中提到"心主身之血脉""主不明则十二官危，使道闭塞而不通，形乃大伤"，表明心的主要功能是化生气血，推动血流在经脉中循行，以濡养全身；而心用以推动全身血流的动力正是心气，心气不足则心不能生化血液，不能维持正常的心搏而致心悸，不能推动血行，血行不利而瘀滞，瘀血阻于脉络，脉络迂曲，"血不利则为水"，继而形成水饮、水肿，即症状进一步加重，心气虚发展为心阳虚的表现。在中医看来，心力衰竭是一个本虚标实的证候，即心气虚导致血瘀继而导致水饮、水肿，心气进一步衰竭而成为心阳虚。

在中医理论中，五脏是一个相互关联的整体，心力衰竭虽病位在心，但也受其他脏腑影响。心气虚，血行不利，化为水，水犯于心，心阳受损，肺脾肾三脏统司一身之水，肺虚不能通调水道，脾虚不能运化水湿，肾虚气化失司，致使水湿停聚，阻滞气机。肺气不畅，肺失宣降，发为喘促；心气不畅，水停于心，则心慌心悸、血行瘀滞，瘀血水饮阻滞；肝气不畅，肝失疏泄，血瘀加重，又加重水肿。

● 心力衰竭的中医治疗方案

对于慢性心力衰竭，中医的诊断主要有以下几种证型及治法方药。

慢性稳定期： ①气虚血瘀证，保元汤合血府逐瘀汤加减，以补益心肺、活血化瘀。②气阴两虚血瘀证，生脉散合血府逐瘀汤加减，以益气养阴、活血化瘀。③阳气虚亏血瘀证，真武汤合血府逐瘀汤加减，以温阳益气、活血化瘀。

急性加重期： ①阳虚水泛证，真武汤合葶苈大枣汤加减，以温阳利水、泻肺平喘。②阳虚喘脱证，以参附龙牡汤回阳固脱。③痰浊壅肺证，以三子养亲汤合真武汤宣肺化痰、蠲饮平喘。

也可选取其他如灸法、穴位贴敷等中医疗法。

心力衰竭的食疗

气虚血瘀证中医药膳食疗方案： 此证型的药膳食疗方主要以健脾益气为主，因此药膳中常用人参、党参、黄芪、山药、茯苓、薏苡仁、芡实等。因人参价高且质优者难求，因此可以党参替代。具体药膳选方有人参三七鸡汤、人参升麻粥、人参茶等。

气阴两虚血瘀证中医药膳食疗方案： 此证型的药膳食疗方主要以益气养阴为主，兼以养心安神，药膳中常用西洋参、党参、黄芪、黄精、山药、百合、麦冬、玉竹等。具体药膳选方有党参淮山薏米煮排骨汤、黄芪西洋参煲鸡汤、莲子百合煲猪瘦肉汤等。

阳虚血瘀证中医药膳食疗方案： 此证型的药膳食疗方

主要以益气温阳为主，药膳中常用红参、黄芪、桂圆、杜仲、冬虫夏草、黑豆、板栗等。具体药膳选方有红参桂圆炖瘦肉汤、黑豆鲤鱼汤、桂圆莲子粥等。

　　其他兼证的中医药膳食疗方案：中、重度心衰患者常伴有水肿的症状，水肿明显者，可予利水渗湿类药膳方，如砂仁鲫鱼汤、鲤鱼赤小豆汤、鲤鱼冬瓜汤、赤小豆冬瓜煲乌鱼、茯苓粳米粥、冬瓜粥、赤小豆茅根汤等。除此之外还有一部分患者伴有严重的失眠，对于失眠者可配合食用酸枣仁粥、小麦红枣粥、安神二枣粥等。

眩晕 ∾
——颈椎病、腰椎病

● 什么是颈椎病、腰椎病?

颈椎病:颈椎病又称颈椎综合征,是颈椎骨关节炎、增生性颈椎炎、颈神经根综合征、颈椎间盘突出症的总称,是一种以退行性病理改变为基础的疾患。主要由于颈椎长期劳损、骨质增生或椎间盘脱出、韧带增厚,致使颈椎脊髓、神经根或椎动脉受压,出现一系列功能障碍的临床综合征。

青少年处于生长发育期,无法用椎间盘退变来解释临床表现。因此,年轻患者出现暂时的颈部不适、影像检查未发现明显退行性病变征象时,不宜急于作出颈椎病的诊断。

腰椎病:腰椎病是腰椎疾病的总称。常见的腰椎疾病主要有腰肌劳损、腰肌筋膜炎、腰椎间盘突出症、腰椎管狭窄症以及脊柱侧凸畸形等疾病,就诊需要到医院的脊柱骨科进行相应的检查,然后根据确诊的结果对症治疗。

为什么会得颈椎病、腰椎病？

颈椎病、腰椎病有的是不良的生活习惯引起的，在平时生活当中，一定要有正确的坐姿和正确的工作姿势，千万不能长期地坐多动少，在感觉身体比较劳累的时候，一定要起身活动，这样才能够预防这些疾病的发生。颈椎病、腰椎病有的是太过劳累引起的，如果长期熬夜，长期坐在电脑面前不动，就会导致颈椎和腰椎受到严重的损伤，久而久之就会导致颈椎病和腰椎病的发生，所以大家一定要学会放松自己。颈椎病、腰椎病有的是不良的饮食习惯引起的，如果在平时生活当中经常吸烟喝酒，经常吃辛辣刺激、过咸、油腻的食物，可能导致颈椎病和腰椎病的发生。

颈椎病、腰椎病有什么症状，对人有什么危害呢？

临床当中颈椎病、腰椎病有很多种类型，不同类型的疾病症状是不一样的。神经根型颈椎病主要是神经根部受到挤压之后产生的，会引起颈部疼痛、上肢的放射性疼痛，也有可能会引起麻木的感觉。脊髓型颈椎病主要是脊髓受到挤压之后产生的，常常会引起双下肢行走不稳，容易摔倒，有脚踩棉花的感觉，双上肢精细动作完成困难。腰椎病，常常是腰椎间盘突出症，椎间盘突出之后会使椎管内的压力产生变化，所以会引起腰痛；也可能会压迫神经根，引起腿部放射性疼痛，或出现麻木的症状。

颈椎病会造成多种危害：颈椎病发生以后，由于患者发病程度、发病时间、个人体质的不同，颈椎病的危害也不尽相同。生活中，多数颈椎病在发病初期症状很轻，不被人们重视，但随着时间的推移，颈椎病患者的病情会不断地恶化。如果颈椎病治疗不及时，引起心理伤害，导致失眠、烦躁、发怒、焦虑、忧郁等症状，将严重危害患者的健康。颈椎病的危害多样，会引起头、颈、肩、背、手臂酸痛，脖子僵硬，活动受限。颈椎病患者的颈肩酸痛，可放射至头枕部和上肢，有的伴有头晕；病情严重的颈椎病患者，甚至会伴有恶心呕吐、卧床不起，少数可有眩晕、猝倒等症状。此外，颈椎病会使得肩背部沉重，上肢无力，手指发麻，肢体皮肤感觉减退，手握物无力，有时不自觉地握物落地。颈椎病的危害还体现在，颈椎病患者会有下肢无力、行走不稳、两脚麻木、行走如踏棉花的感觉。当颈椎病累及交感神经时，患者会出现头晕、头痛、视力模糊、两眼发胀发干、眼睛睁不开、耳鸣、耳堵甚至胃肠胀气等症状。

腰椎病会造成多种危害：①腰痛，95%以上的腰椎病患者有此症状。一种为患者自觉腰部持续性钝痛，平卧时减轻，站立则加剧，一般情况下尚可忍受，可适度活动腰部或慢步行走；另一种为突发的腰部痉挛样剧痛，难以忍受，需卧床休息，严重影响生活和工作。②下肢放射痛，

80%患者出现此症，常在腰痛减轻或消失后出现。表现为由腰部至大腿及小腿后侧的放射性刺激或麻木感，直达足底部。重者可为由腰至足部的电击样剧痛，且多伴有麻木感。疼痛轻者可行走，呈跛行状态；重者需卧床休息，喜欢屈腰、屈髋、屈膝位。③下肢麻木、发冷及间歇性跛行。下肢麻木多与疼痛伴发，少数患者可表现为单纯麻木或自觉下肢发冷、发凉。④马尾神经症状，主要见于中央型髓核脱出症，临床上较少见。可出现会阴部麻木、刺痛，大小便功能障碍，严重者可出现大小便失控及双下肢不完全性瘫痪。

🔵 得了颈椎病、腰椎病该怎么吃？

颈椎病、腰椎病患者的饮食原则为：合理搭配，不可单一偏食。颈椎病、腰椎病患者的膳食一般分为两大类：一类是主食，主要是提供热量，如米、面；另一类食物，可以调节生理机能，称为副食，如豆类、水果和蔬菜等。不同的主食中所含的营养是不同的，粗细要同时吃，不可单一偏食。粗细、干稀、主副搭配的全面营养可满足人体需要，促进患者的康复。

由于颈椎病、腰椎病是椎体增生或骨质退化疏松等引起的，所以颈椎病、腰椎病患者应以富含钙、蛋白质、维生素B族和维生素E的饮食为主。其中钙是骨的主要成分，以牛奶、鱼、猪尾骨、黄豆、黑豆等含量为多；蛋白质是形成韧带、骨骼、肌肉所不可缺少的营养素；维生素B、维生素E则可缓解疼痛和疲劳。

颈椎病如属湿热阻滞经络者，应多吃葛根、苦瓜、丝瓜等清热解肌通络的果蔬；如属寒湿阻滞经络者，应多吃狗肉、羊肉等温经散寒的食物；如属血虚气滞者，应多吃公鸡、鲤鱼、黑豆等食物。

总之，对证对症进食，有利于颈椎病、腰椎病患者的康复。视力模糊、流泪者，宜多食含钙、硒、锌的食物，如豆制品、动物肝脏、蛋、鱼、蘑菇、芦笋、胡萝卜等；颈椎病伴高血压者，宜多吃豆芽、海带、木耳、大蒜、芹菜、地瓜、冬瓜、绿豆等。颈椎病、腰椎病患者最好戒烟酒，不要经常吃生冷和过热的食物，忌油腻厚味之品，忌辛辣刺激性食物。

● 得了颈椎病、腰椎病该怎么运动？

平时注意坐姿，避免颈椎过度劳损，避免枕过高的枕头，适当锻炼颈背肌，包括颈部的转动、双肩关节的活动。在工间或工余时，做头及双上肢的前屈、后伸及旋转运动，既可缓解疲劳，又能使肌肉发达、韧度增强，从而有利于颈段脊柱的稳定性，增强颈肩顺应颈部突然变化的能力。有氧运动能减轻腰椎负担，还能有效增强腰椎柔韧性和肌肉力量，可以有效缓解以及预防腰痛的症状。适宜的有氧运动主要有：快走或慢跑、骑自行车、登山和退步走等。

快走或慢跑：做这两项运动时建议穿有弹性的运动

鞋，抬头挺胸，每天大约活动半个小时，一般腰椎术后患者建议适量步行，通常腰肌劳损等退行性腰椎病患者要有适量的活动时间，但不要过量运动，避免过于劳累。

骑自行车：患者在骑车时车座应尽量降低一点，把手调高一点，骑车一般对腰椎管狭窄患者比较有利，它能增加腰椎管宽度和腰椎柔韧性，每天可坚持运动半个小时左右，对于腰椎有很好的改善作用。

登山运动：登山一般能锻炼大腿肌肉和腰肌力量，要适量锻炼，建议不要过度劳累，以免增加腰椎负担。在登山时建议避免斜坡角度大的山路，有意让腹肌用力，能让膝关节稍微屈曲，对腰椎有很好的改善作用。

退步走：患者可每天退步走大约50分钟，但要以不加重症状为度，建议走的时候尽可能往后倒，一般走完后会微感疲劳。

💬 得了颈椎病、腰椎病该怎么治疗？

颈椎病和腰椎病是现代人群中常见的关节疾病，大多是由于久坐、长时间伏案工作、长时间玩手机电脑导致的，一般很难完全治愈，只能通过调整日常生活方式进行缓解。颈椎病患者不要长时间伏案，适当进行颈部活动和按摩，可以外敷一些活血化瘀的膏药，例如金黄膏，同时要注意保暖；腰椎疾病患者不要久站久坐，女性要少穿高跟鞋，睡觉时床板不要过软，适当进行烤电治疗和外敷膏药配以中医手法按摩。

颈椎病、腰椎病的治疗，首先应该去正规医院检查清楚。诊断明确是颈椎间盘或腰椎间盘严重突出，还是轻微的膨出。诊断明确后，在病情不严重的情况下，可以通过纠正不良姿势，比如久坐久站、长期弯腰负重或低头伏案工作、玩手机；同时进行颈椎和腰椎的适当锻炼，比如三点、五点支撑锻炼，并配合药物、物理理疗进行保守治疗。治疗颈椎病和腰椎病，最好是保守治疗，可以做局部的推拿按摩，促进局部的血液循环，缓解颈椎和腰椎局部肌肉紧张的情况。腰椎疼痛要注意休息，睡觉尽量睡硬板床；而颈椎疼痛要注意运动，需多活动颈椎关节。如果颈椎间盘、腰椎间盘突出比较严重，压迫神经脊髓，引起肌肉无力、活动受限的情况，就需要采取手术治疗。

🔵 中医是怎么认识颈椎病、腰椎病的？

虽然在中医学中并无"颈椎病""腰椎间盘突出"等关于颈椎、腰椎疾病的病名，但中医学早就有关于其症状的论述，散见于"痹证""颈项强痛""颈肩痛""腰脊痛""腰腿痛"等疾病中，所述内容涉及了颈腰椎疾病的病因、病机、病位和治疗等各个方面。

《素问·痹论》曰："风寒湿三气杂至，合而为痹也。其风气胜者为行痹，寒气胜者为痛痹，湿气胜者为着痹也。"《素问·至真要大论》称"诸痉项强，皆属于湿""湿淫所胜……病冲头痛，目似脱，项似拔"，其发病及症状特点与颈椎病相似。《素问·长刺节论》

常见心血管病相关科普知识

081

称："病在骨，骨重不可举，骨髓酸痛，寒气至，名曰骨痹。"《景岳全书·杂证谟·湿证》："湿之为病，……在经络则为痹，为重，为筋骨疼痛，为腰痛不能转侧，为四肢痿弱酸痛……"在东汉时期，张仲景就认识到了五六十岁的中老年人，由于劳损易患颈椎病。他在《金匮要略》中指出："人年五六十，其病脉大者，痹挟背行，若肠鸣、马刀、侠瘿者，皆为劳得之。"《东垣试效方·腰痛论》："足太阳膀胱之脉所过，还出别下项，循肩膊内，挟脊抵腰中，故为病者项如拔，挟脊痛，腰似折，髀不可以曲，是经气虚则邪客之，痛病生矣。"《医学心悟》："腰痛拘急，牵引腿足。"总之，有关颈椎、腰椎疾病症状的论述甚多，体现古代医家对此类认识的多重性，也说明本病在古代文献中所涉及范围的广泛性。

颈椎病、腰椎病的病因病机，可以概括为以下三个方面。①肝肾亏损，筋脉失养。中医学认为肾主骨生髓，肝主筋藏血，且肝肾同源，故颈椎病、腰椎病与肝肾关系最为密切。肾精充则骨髓充盈，骨骼得以滋养，方强劲坚固，动作敏捷；肝有所藏以养五脏六腑、四肢百骸，筋得血养则强健有力。肝肾亏虚则髓空精少，筋骨失养而致筋骨不坚，经络不畅而发为颈肩腰腿痛。②跌仆闪挫，气血瘀滞。脏腑机能衰退，肝肾亏虚，髓空精少，四肢百骸失之荣养，而致筋骨不坚，易受损伤。特别是长期劳累过度，或有跌仆坠堕，损及肌肉筋脉，导致脉络痹阻，气血瘀滞，不通则痛。《景岳全书》曰："跌仆伤而腰痛者，此伤在筋骨，而血脉凝滞也。"③寒湿内侵，阻遏经络。中老年人年高体衰，脏腑机能衰退，肝肾亏虚，气血不足，卫外不固，风寒湿邪易乘虚而入，内侵经脉，阻滞气血，肾府更失所荣，不荣则痛。《素问·痹论》说："风寒湿三气杂至，合而为痹也。"《素问·举痛论》说："寒气入经而稽迟，泣而不行，客于脉外则血少，客于脉中则气不通，故卒然而痛。"

颈椎病、腰椎病的中医治疗方案

中医学认为腰椎间盘突出症的主要病机在于"不通则痛"和"不荣则痛"两个方面。根据"实则泻之，虚则补之"的基本治疗原则，临床上对于该病的治疗也应该以"补法"和"通法"为主。补法重在滋补肝肾、强筋壮骨；通法以活血化瘀、通络止痛、清热除湿、温散寒湿等为主。对于临床表现为虚实夹杂证的患者，则应根据感受邪气的不同以及气血阴阳亏虚的不同，运用"通补兼施"的治疗方法，"泻实不忘补虚，补虚不忘泻实"，"通法"与"补法"应当相互配合使用。在临证时应审证求因、辨证施治，根据患者不同情况选取方药。

颈椎病、腰椎病的食疗

根据患者的病情，为患者制订不同的中医食疗方案。风寒湿痹者，可食用大蒜、羊肉、胡椒根等；气滞血瘀者，可食用山楂丹参粥；上肢麻木者，可食用葛根猪骨汤。

附 录

调养功法（英文版）

Antihypertensive and Sleep Assist Exercise

(For alleviating hypertension and improving sleep)

This exercise aims to regulate blood pressure and improve the quality of sleep. It is based on the theories of Traditional Chinese Medicine(TCM), acupuncture and tuina as well as the author's practice and study for several years. In this exercise, various manipulations such as pressing, kneading, twisting, pushing, stroking, rubbing are basic techniques to harmonize yin and yang, regulate qi-activity, pacify liver while restraining yang and nourish liver and kidney, through which you can get a comprehensive whole-body movement to improve qi and blood circulation. Therefore, it can be applied to treat primary hypertension, insomnia, headache, vertigo, depression, anxiety, climacteric syndrome and many other related diseases.

The body can be divided into three parts: the head-neck part, the torso-and-upper-limb part and the lower-limb part. This exercise focuses on the head-neck part, while exercise of the other parts helps reinforce the curative effect. The mainly

🌓 Step 1

Press and knead Baihui (GV20) to refresh your mind

✏ Body: Raise your left arm and press Baihui(GV20) acupoint with your left hypothenar six times evenly. Then change pressing into kneading around the same point counterclockwise. Next, put your left arm down and raise your right arm to take the same manipulations. The difference is that you are supposed to knead around Baihui(GV20) clockwise with your right hypothenar. Alternate left and right arms and repeat six times. (Picture2, Picture3)

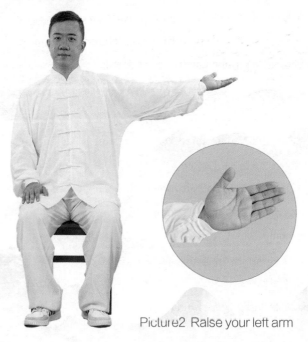

Picture2 Raise your left arm

常见心血管病调养功法

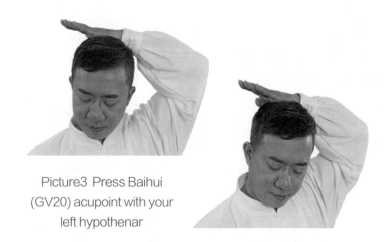

Picture3 Press Baihui
(GV20) acupoint with your
left hypothenar

    ⌒ Breath: Exhale when you use strength to press and inhale when not. Slow down your breath when you knead Baihui(GV20). Do not knead too fast. When you take one breath, you just knead a circle.

    ⌒ Meditation:Try to have meditation without distractions. Concentrate your mind on the lower dantian.

⌒ Functional effect ⌒

    Baihui, alias "three Yang five Hui". It belongs to the governor vessel. Located in the head, the front hairline is straight up 5 cun. Indications: headache, dizziness, nasal congestion, tinnitus, stroke, aphasia, etc. Pressing and kneading Baihui, can play the role of enlightening the body and awakening the brain, and has a good improvement effect on dizziness, headache and other symptoms common in patients with hypertension.

Step 2

Press and knead Fengchi(GB20) to refresh ears and eyes

🍃 Body: Hold your hands behind the head. Then put thumbs into Fengchi(GB20) acupoints at both sides, loose palm against the head. Press the acupoints six times evenly. Next, knead the same points with your left thumb counterclockwise and right clockwise together six times. Rest a while and repeat four times. (Picture4, Picture5)

🍃 Breath: Exhale when you use strength to press and inhale when not. Slow down your breath when you knead. Do not knead too fast. When you take one breath, you just knead a circle.

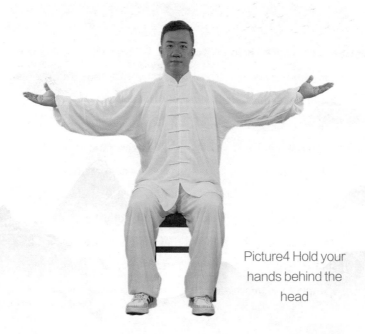

Picture4 Hold your hands behind the head

附录 调养功法（英文版）

091

常见心血管病调养功法

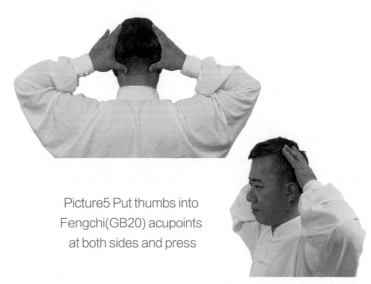

Picture5 Put thumbs into
Fengchi(GB20) acupoints
at both sides and press

⤢ Meditation: Try to have meditation without distractions. Concentrate your mind on the lower dantian.

⤢ Functional effect ⤢

Fengchi belongs to the foot Shaoyang gallbladder meridian, which is the intersection of foot Shaoyang gallbladder meridian and yang link vessel. In the nape, below the occipital bone, level with the Fengfu, in the depression between the sternocleidomastoid and the upper end of the trapezius. Treating headache, dizziness, fever and cold, eye swelling pain, tinnitus, deafness, etc. Pressing and kneading Fengchi can play the role of calming the liver to stop the wind and promoting the circulation of organs and orifice, and have a good effect on improving the head symptoms of patients with hypertension and insomnia.

☯ Step 3

Press and knead Yingxiang(LI20) to relieve your stuffy nose

✎ Body: Both hands are in the shape of "V", and the index fingers of both hands slide down from Yintang(EX-HN3) point to press Jingming(BL1) point and Yingxiang(LI20) point . Next, knead the same points with your left index finger counterclockwise and right clockwise together six times. Repeat four times. (From Picture6 to Picture8)

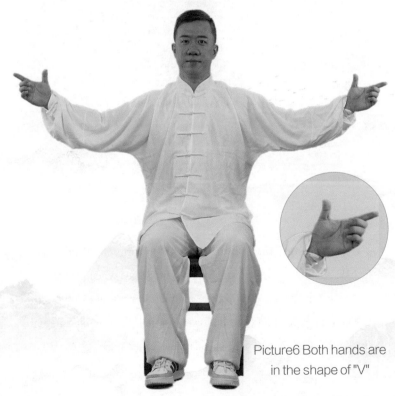

Picture6 Both hands are
in the shape of "V"

附录 调养功法（英文版）

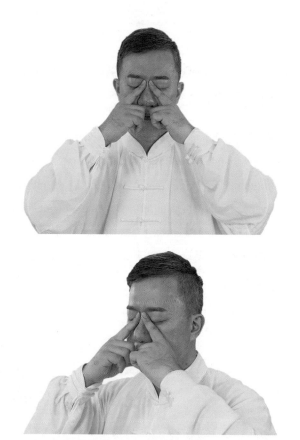

Picture7 The index fingers of both hands slide down from
Yintang (EX-HN3)

         Breath: Take normal respiration throughout this step.
Exhale when you use strength to press and inhale when not.

         Meditation: Try to have meditation without distractions.
Concentrate your mind on the lower dantian. Imagine an internal
flow going from Yintang(EX-HN3) down to the nose.

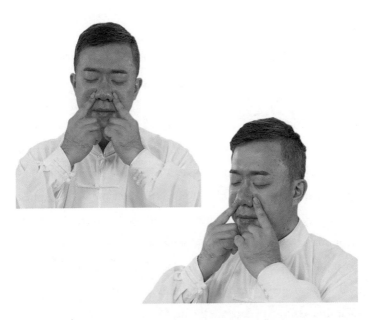

Picture8 Press Yingxiang(LI20) acupoints

❧ Functional effect ❧

Yingxiang belongs to the large intestine meridian of hand Yangming. This acupoint is beside the middle point of the outer edge of the nasal alar, located in the nasolabial groove. It has the function of evacuating wind-heat and promoting nasal orifices opening, mainly used in the treatment of nasal congestion, epistaxis, crooked mouth, and other diseases. Rubbing Yingxiang can relieve stuffy nose and smooth breathing, and has a good effect on improving the symptoms of patients with hypertension and insomnia.

🌀 Step 4

Press Taiyang(EX-HN5) along the head laterals to alleviate your headache

✑ Body: Make your fingers like a "sword" (i.e. bend your ring and little fingers, so that your index and middle fingers can be straight out in parallel just like a sword). Use your index and middle fingers to press both Touwei(ST8) acupoints six times. Then go down slowly to knead around both Taiyang(EX-HN5) acupoints, left hand counterclockwise(right hand clockwise). Next, go down and compress the edge of the ears with your thumb and index fingers. Finally, pinch your earlobes six times. Repeat four times.(From Picture9 to Picture14)

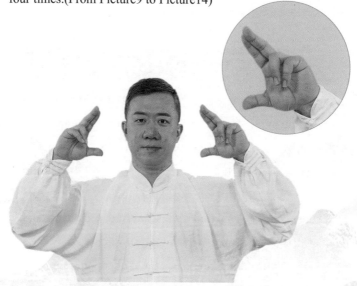

Picture9 Make your fingers like a "sword"

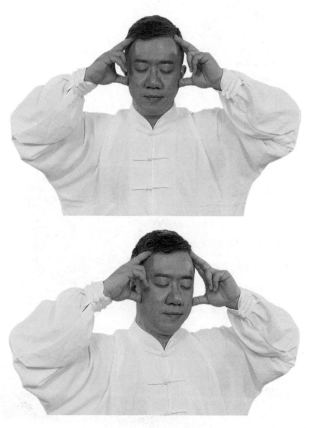

Picture10 Press both Touwei(ST8) acupoints

   ◡ Breath: Take normal respiration throughout this step. Exhale when you use strength to press and inhale when not. Breathe evenly and naturally.

   ◡ Meditation: Try to have meditation without distractions. Concentrate your mind on the lower dantian. Imagine an internal flow going from Taiyang(EX-HN5) acupoints down to the earlobes.

附
录
调养功法（英文版）

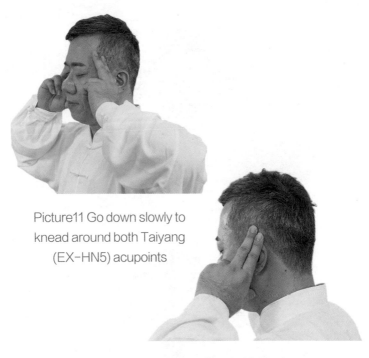

Picture11 Go down slowly to knead around both Taiyang (EX-HN5) acupoints

Picture12 Go down

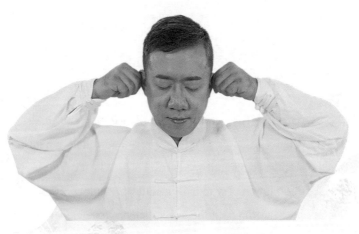

Picture13 Go down and compress the edge of the ears with your thumb and index fingers

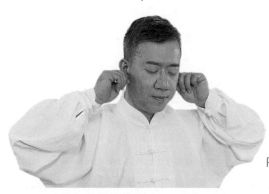

Picture14 Pinch
your earlobes

Touwei is the acupoint of the foot Yangming stomach meridian, which is the intersection of foot Yangming stomach meridian, foot Shaoyang gall bladder meridian and yang link vessel. Located in the frontal angle 0.5 cun above the hairline, beside the median line of the head, 4.5 cun away from the Shenting, in the galea aponeurotica of the upper margin of the temporal muscle. The indications are headache, dizziness, eye pain, windward tears and other diseases. Taiyang is located on either side of the forehead, the outer upper part of the eye socket, extending to the upper edge of the ear. Taiyang has the effect of clearing heat for detumescence, relieving pain and relieving collaterals, and can treat migraine, dizziness, mouth and eye skew and other diseases. Sequential rubbing Touwei, Taiyang and earlobe, can comprehensively adjust the head symptoms of patients with hypertension and insomnia, such as headache, dizziness, and blurred vision.

附录 调养功法（英文版）

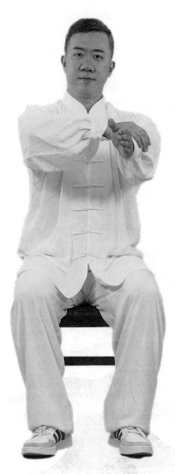

☯ Step 5
Rub hand-meridians to relax your arms

✐ Body: Raise your left arm in front of chest. Put your right thumb on the inside lateral of your left upper arm and the other fingers outside. Use your thumb to rub from upwards to downwards along the pericardium meridian inside while using the other fingers to rub along the large intestine meridian outside. When it comes to Shousanli(LI10), Neiguan(PC6) and Hegu(LI4) acupoints, your fingers should be used to press those acupoints three times respectively. Alternate left and right hands and repeat four times. (From Picture15 to Picture17)

Picture15 Put your right thumb on the inside lateral of your left upper arm and the other fingers outside

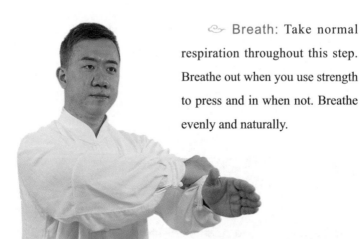

Picture16 Use your thumb to rub from upwards to downwards along the pericardium meridian inside while using the other fingers to rub along the large intestine meridian outside, and press the Shousanli(LI10) , Neiguan(PC6) acupoints

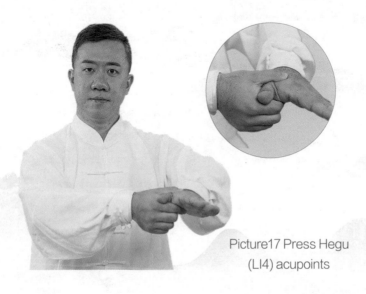

Picture17 Press Hegu (LI4) acupoints

附录 调养功法（英文版）

101

› Meditation: Try to have meditation without distractions. Concentrate your mind on the lower dantian. Look straight ahead and imagine a flow of qi from your shoulders to your fingertips along both sides of your arms.

∾ Functional effect ∾

Acupoints of Jueyin pericardium meridian of hand are mainly used to treat heart, chest, stomach, mental diseases, and other diseases in the place where the meridians follow. The treatment of heart, chest and stomach diseases commonly used Quze, Ximen, Jianshi, Neiguan and Daling; the treatment of mental diseases commonly used Jianshi, Laogong, Zhongchong. Neiguan has the effect of raising and floating Sanjiao, waking up the brain to open the orifices, moving qi to relieve pain; Tianchi is mainly used to treat chest pain and cardiopulmonary disease. The main acupoints on the large intestine meridian treat diseases of the head, facial features and throat, mental diseases, fever and other diseases on the meridian route. By pressing the external and internal channels at the same time, the corresponding meridian points can be comprehensively stimulated, and the cardiothoracic discomfort of patients with hypertension and insomnia can be improved, which has a good symptom improvement effect.

🌓 Step 6

Press and knead Danzhong(CV17) to promote the circulation of cardiac vessels

✍ Body: Put your left hypothenar on Danzhong(CV17) and press six times. Then knead the same point counterclockwise six times. Alternate left and right hands and repeat four times. (Picture 18)

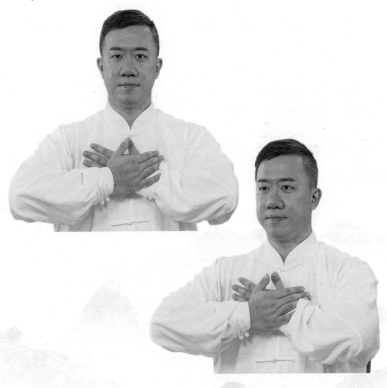

Picture18 Put your left hypothenar on Danzhong(CV17)
and press, then knead the same point

  ✑ Breath: Take normal respiration throughout this step. Breathe out when you use strength to press or knead and in when not. Breathe evenly and naturally.

  ✑ Meditation: Try to have meditation without distractions. Concentrate your mind on the lower dantian. Close your eyes slightly and imagine that the qi stagnation inside your chest gradually disperses.

✑ Functional effect ✑

Danzhong belongs to the conception vessel, located in the anterior median line, flat between the fourth rib, the midpoint of the connection between the two nipples, on the sternal body. Indications of asthma, chest pain, palpitation, upset and other symptoms. Rubbing Danzhong, can alleviate hypertension, insomnia patients with chest tightness, pain or palpitation and other symptoms.

☯ Step 7

Rub Shenshu(BL23) to keep your body warm

✑ Body: Use your palms to press Shenshu(BL23) acupoints on the bladder meridian. Rub downwards along the bladder meridian from Shenshu(BL23) to Guanyuanshu(BL26). Repeat six times to make your renal regions feel a little warmer. (Picture19, Picture20)

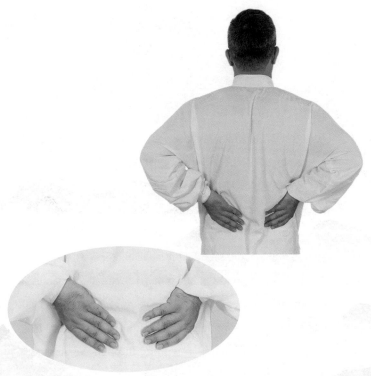

Picture19 Use your palms to press Shenshu(BL23) acupoints on the bladder meridian

常见心血管病调养功法

◦ Breath: Exhale when rubbing downwards and inhale during the interval. Breathe evenly and naturally.

◦ Meditation: Try to have meditation without distractions. Concentrate on your lower dantian. Close your eyes slightly and imagine warm flows streaming inside your renal regions.

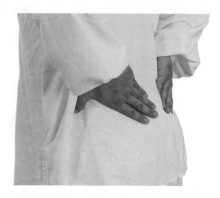

Picture20 Rub downwards along the bladder meridian to Guanyuanshu(BL26)

◦ Functional effect ◦

Shenshu is one of the commonly used points on the foot Taiyang bladder meridian.It is located under the spinous process of the second lumbar spine, 1.5 cun apart, between the lumbar dorsal fascia, longissimus muscle and iliocostal muscle. Indications are lumbago, tinnitus and deafness. This set of exercises from top to bottom, through the stroke of Shenshu to tonifying kidney qi, filling essence and tonifying the brain.

☯ Step 8

Press acupoints on the spleen and kidney meridians to nourish your brain

✐ Body: Use both hands to rub from the central thighs downwards to the feet. When meeting Xuehai(SP10), Zusanli(ST36) and Sanyinjiao(SP6), your fingers should be used to press those acupoints six times respectively. Repeat four times. (From Picture21 to Picture23)

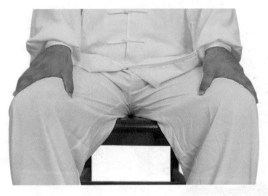

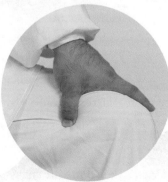

Picture21 Press Xuehai (SP10) acupoints

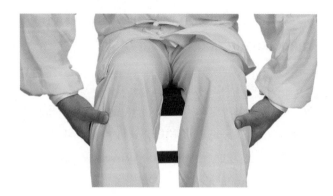

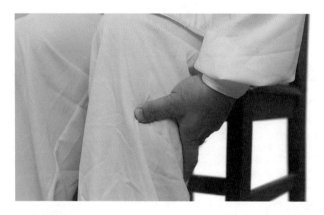

Picture22 Press Zusanli(ST36) acupoints

    ᠅ Breath: Exhale when rubbing downwards and inhale during the interval. Breathe evenly and naturally.

    ᠅ Meditation: Try to have meditation without distractions. Concentrate on your lower dantian. Close your eyes slightly. Imagine warm flows streaming inside from thigh to toes.

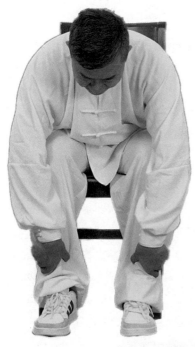

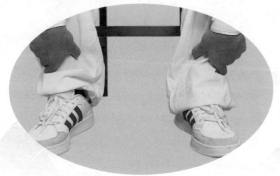

Picture23 Press Sanyinjiao(SP6) acupoints

✎ Functional effect ✎

Zusanli is one of the main acupoints of the foot Yangming stomach meridian. It is located on the outside of the calf, 3 cun below Dubi, and on the line between Dubi and Jiexi. It is used to treat gastrointestinal disease syndrome, lower limb atrophy syndrome, mental disease, surgical disease, syndrome of exhaustion. Sanyinjiao is one of the commonly used acupoints of the foot Taiyin spleen meridian. It is the intersection point of the three yin meridians of foot(liver, spleen and kidney), which is located on the medial side of the calf, 3 cun above the tip of the medial ankle of the foot, and behind the medial edge of the tibia. Often kneading this point can adjust and tonify the liver, spleen and kidney's qi and blood, the treatment of endocrine disorders, hypertension, diabetes, coronary heart disease are significant. Xuehai, knee flexion in the inner thigh, 2 cun above the medial end of the bottom of the patella, when the bulge of the medial head of the quadriceps femoris. Xuehai is to generate blood and promote blood stasis. Pressing and kneading these three acupoints, can regulate the liver and kidney, promote qi and blood circulation.

🜨 Step 9

Press Taichong(LR3) to regulate qi

✍ Body: Put your left leg on the right thigh. Then use your right thumb to press Taichong(LR3) six times to feel a little sore. Next, use your left thumb to knead Yongquan(KI1) counterclockwise six times to feel a little sore. Alternate left and right feet and repeat four times. (Picture24, Picture25)

✍ Breath: Take normal respiration throughout this step. Exhale when you use strength to press or knead and inhale when not. Breathe evenly and naturally.

✍ Meditation: Try to have meditation without distractions. Concentrate your mind on the lower dantian.

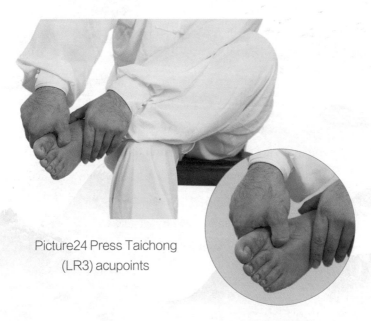

Picture24 Press Taichong
(LR3) acupoints

附录 调养功法（英文版）

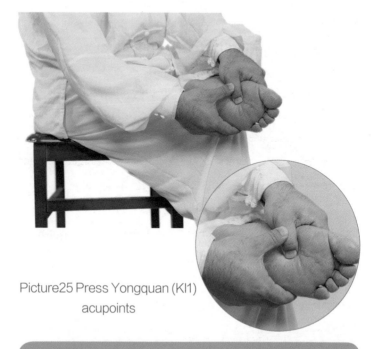

Picture25 Press Yongquan (KI1)
acupoints

✑ Functional effect ✑

Taichong belongs to the foot Jueyin liver meridian, located on the dorsum of the foot, between the first and second metatarsal bones, the anterior depression of the junction of the base of the metatarsal bone. It has the effect of soothing the liver and regulating qi, clearing the liver and gall bladder, clearing the heat and reducing the fire, pacifying liver and subduing yang, dredging channels and activating collaterals. Through the point pressure of Taichong, it can relieve the symptoms of headache and dizziness, soothing the liver and relieving depression.

Closing posture

Sit down with eyes closed in tranquility. Tighten up the belly and harbour the chest. Relax your legs and put your palms on the thighs. Breathe evenly so that you can slowly swallow your saliva at the same time. After three minutes, it is finished to stand up.

附录 调养功法（英文版）

常见心血管病调养功法

Cardiac Insufficiency
Regulation Exercise
(For tonifying qi and strengthening your body)

This exercise aims at improving the health condition of people suffering from heart failure and asthenia. It is based on the theories of TCM, acupuncture and tuina as well as the author's practice and study for several years. In this exercise, various manipulations such as pressing, kneading, rubbing, are basic techniques. The movement of qi and blood is regulated by stimulation of local acupoints and small range of body movements, to achieve the purpose of supplementing yang, nourishing yin and activating blood to relieve edema. Therefore, it can be applied to treat heart failure, asthenia, chronic fatigue syndrome(CFS) and many other related diseases.

The body can be divided into three parts: the head-neck part, the torso-and-upper-limb part and the lower-limb part. This exercise focuses on the torso-and-upper-limb part, while exercise of the other parts helps reinforce the curative effect. The mainly stimulated acupoints of the head-neck part are Baihui(GV20) and Yintang(EX-HN3). The mainly stimulated acupoints of the torso-and-upper-limb part are Neiguan(PC6), Danzhong(CV17), Guanyuan(CV4), Zhongji(CV3) and Qihai(CV6). The mainly stimulated acupoints of the lower-limb part are Zusanli(ST36), Sanyinjiao(SP6) and Yongquan(KI1).

Sequence of the exercise: from head to toe and left to right.

☯ Opening posture

Both lying and sitting postures are viable. Let's take the sitting posture as an example.

✍ Body: Total body relaxation. Sit on the chair with your eyes gently closed, tongue against the palate and lips overlapped slightly. Put your arms loose beside your side and separate your feet in line with your shoulders. (Picture 26)

✍ Breath: Breathe naturally. Calm down. Take abdominal respiration.

✍ Meditation: Relax your mind. Concentrate your mind on the lower dantian.

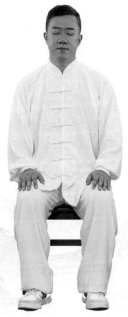

Picture26 Opening posture

☯ Step 1

Tongue against palate in quiet state to tonify qi and yin

◈ Body: Reach your tongue to the palate and use a little strength to press six times. Wait for five seconds. Then repeat four times. Finally, swallow your accumulating saliva slowly. (Picture 27)

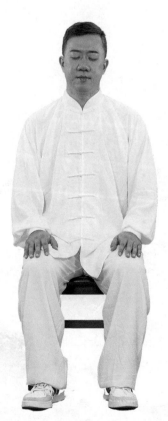

Picture27 Reach your tongue to the palate and use a little strength to press

附录 调养功法 (英文版)

常见心血管病调养功法

 Breath: Breathe out when you use strength to press and in when not. Take normal respiration throughout this step, Not too fast. Press once when you just take a whole breath.

 Meditation: Try to have meditation without distractions. Concentrate your mind on the lower dantian.

☜ Functional effect ☞

Fluid in the mouth is produced by the tongue against the upper palate in step1, TCM believes that it has the effect of nourishing yin and tonifying kidney. Practice has proved that it can relieve the symptoms of dry mouth and bitter taste in mouth.

Step 2

Press Yintang(EX-HN3) to refresh your mind and eyes

 Body: Raise your hands and make your two index fingers like an inverted type of "V". Then use your two index fingers to press Yintang(EX-HN3) six times alternatively. Next, use your index fingers to knead Yintang(EX-HN3), left index finger clockwise, right index finger counterclockwise six times. Repeat four times. (Picture28)

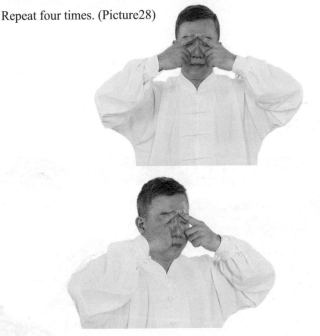

Picture28 Make your two index fingers like an inverted type of "V" to press and knead Yintang(EX-HN3)

附录　调养功法（英文版）

      ⌘ Breath: Take normal respiration throughout this step. Breathe out when you use strength to press and in when not.

      ⌘ Meditation: Try to have meditation without distractions. Concentrate your mind on the lower dantian. Imagine a piece of qi accumulating inside Yintang(EX-HN3).

⌘ Functional effect ⌘

      Yintang belongs to the extra point. This acupoint is located on the forehead of the human body, in the middle of the two eyebrows. It has the effect of brightening the eyes, clearing the nose and calming the mind. It is mainly used in the clinical treatment of insomnia, headache and other symptoms. Pressing Yingtang can improve the sleep of patients with cardiac insufficiency and relieve the symptoms such as headache.

Step 3

Press and knead conception vessel(CV6) to elevate yang qi

   Body: Use your overlapped palms to press the belly between Guanyuan(CV4) and Qihai(CV6) six times to feel a little warmer in the middle of your hand. Then knead where you press previously counterclockwise six times to feel a little warmer inside your belly. Repeat four times.(Picture29)

   Breath: Exhale when you use strength to press or knead and inhale when not. Breathe evenly and naturally throughout this step.

   Meditation: Try to have meditation without distractions, close your eyes. Concentrate your mind on the lower dantian, where you should imagine warm flows streaming inside.

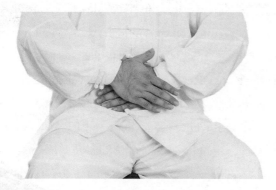

Picture29 Use your overlapped palms to press the belly between Guanyuan (CV4) and Qihai(CV6)，then knead where you press previously

附录 调养功法（英文版）

✑ **Functional effect** ✑

Guanyuan belongs to the conception vessel, which is the intersection point of foot three yin meridians and conception vessel. It is the front-mu point of small intestines. Lower abdomen, anterior median line, 3 cun below the umbilicus. Indications for apoplexy, kidney deficiency and asthma, spermatorrhea, impotence, hernia, enuresis, dripping, urinary frequency, urinary occlusion, uterine prolapse, neurasthenia, syncope, shock, etc. It has a strong effect. Qihai belongs to the conception vessel, which is the original point of Huang. Lower abdomen, anterior median line, 1.5 cun below the umbilicus. It is used for the treatment of prostration, syncope, abdominal pain, diarrhea, menstrual disorder, dysmenorrhea, uterine bleeding, prolapse, spermatorrhea, impotence, enuresis, hernia and urinary retention, urinary tract infection, intestinal obstruction, etc. and has a strong effect. Guanyuan and Qihai are the classic acupoints of TCM, which can supplement qi and blood and warm yang qi. Rubbing or moxibustion has a good clinical effect, which can improve many debilitating symptoms such as weakness, fatigue, and sexual function decline in patients with cardiac insufficiency.

☯ Step 4

Press Zusanli(ST36) to reinforce the spleen and stomach

✍ Body: Use your thumbs to press Zusanli(ST36) acupoints six times, then left thumb counterclockwise and right thumb clockwise knead the same points six times. Repeat four times. (Picture30)

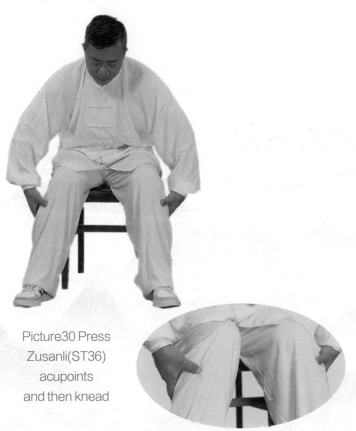

Picture30 Press
Zusanli(ST36)
acupoints
and then knead

附录 调养功法（英文版）

  Breath: Exhale when you use strength to press and inhale when not. Breathe evenly and naturally.

  Meditation: Try to have meditation without distractions. Concentrate your mind on the lower dantian. Close your eyes and imagine warm flows gathering inside Zusanli(ST36) acupoints.

∂ Functional effect ∂

Zusanli is one of the main acupoints of the foot Yangming stomach meridian. It is located on the outside of the calf, 3 cun below Dubi, and on the line between Dubi and Jiexi. It is used to treat gastrointestinal disease syndrome, lower limb atrophy syndrome, mental disease, surgical disease, syndrome of exhaustion. As a classic strong point in traditional Chinese medicine, Zusanli has the effect of tonifying spleen and qi, strengthening and tonifying deficiency. By kneading and persisting for a long time, it has a good effect on improving the weakness symptoms in patients with cardiac insufficiency.

🏵 Step 5

Press Sanyinjiao(SP6) to replenish fluid

✍ Body: Put your right leg on the left thing. Use your thumbs to press Sanyinjiao(SP6) six times, then left thumb counterclockwise and right thumb clockwise knead the same points six times. Alternate left and right feet and repeat four times. (Picture31)

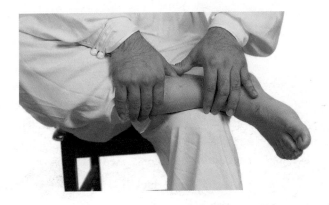

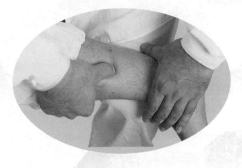

Picture31 Press Sanyinjiao(SP6) acupoints and then knead

常见心血管病调养功法

  Breath: Exhale when you use strength to press or knead and inhale when not. Breathe evenly and naturally.

  Meditation: Try to have meditation without distractions. Concentrate your mind on the lower dantian. Close your eyes and imagine warm flows gathering inside Sanyinjiao(SP6) acupoints.

✑ Functional effect ✑

Sanyinjiao is one of the commonly used acupoints of the foot Taiyin spleen meridian, which is the intersection point of the three yin meridians of foot (liver, spleen and kidney). It is located on the medial side of the calf, 3 cun above the tip of the medial ankle of the foot, and behind the medial edge of the tibia. Often kneading this point can adjust the liver, spleen, kidney's qi and blood. By kneading, long-term adherence has a good effect on improving the symptoms of liver and kidney yin deficiency in patients with cardiac insufficiency.

Step 6

Press and knead Yongquan(KI1) to regulate qi

▸ Body: Put your right leg on the left thigh. Then use your right thumb to press Yongquan(KI1) acupoint on your left foot to feel a little distending sore. Next, knead the same point six times. Alternate left and right feet and repeat four times. (Picture32)

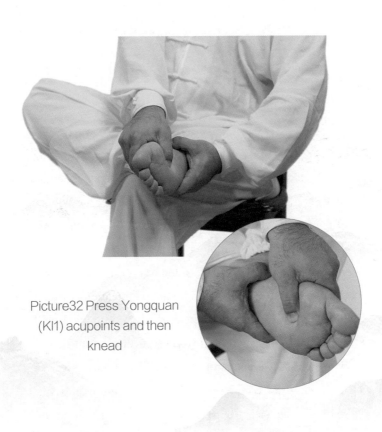

Picture32 Press Yongquan (KI1) acupoints and then knead

附录 调养功法（英文版）

☞ Breath: Exhale when you use strength to press or knead and inhale when not. Breathe evenly and naturally.

☞ Meditation: Try to have meditation without distractions. Concentrate your mind on the lower dantian. Imagine qi gathering inside Yongquan(KI1) acupoints.

☞ Functional effect ☞

Yongquan is one of the commonly used points on the foot Shaoyin kidney meridian. It is located at the bottom of the foot, in the depression of the front of the foot when the foot is curled, about the intersection of the first 1/3 and second 2/3 of the line between the head of the second and third plantar toe suture and the heel. Indications of lung disease, constipation, inhibited urination, running piglet. Kneading Yongquan can promote urination and stool pass, nourish yin and tonify kidney, it has a good effect on improving the symptoms of fu-qi obstruction and liver-kidney yin deficiency in patients with cardiac insufficiency.

Closing posture

Sit down with your eyes closed in tranquility. Chest adduction and abdomen in. Separate your legs and put your hands alongside naturally. Breathe evenly so that you can swallow your saliva slowly. After five minutes, it is finished to get up.

常见心血管病调养功法

Vertigo Regulation Exercise
(For improving spinal structure and function)

This exercise aims at improving the physical condition of patients suffering from cervical spondylosis, scapulohumeral periarthritis and relieving the pain in the neck, shoulder, waist and leg. It is based on the theories of TCM, acupuncture and tuina as well as the author's practice and study for several years. This exercise is mainly based on local joint rotation and whole-body movement. During this exercise, through which you can relax your sinews, activate blood and regulate sinew-and-bone function. Therefore, it can be applied to treat cervical spondylosis, scapulohumeral periarthritis, the pain in the neck, shoulder, waist and leg, etc.

This set of exercises divides the position of the human body into three parts: head and neck, upper body and lower limbs. Head and neck movements are the main focus, supplemented by trunk and upper limbs, lower limbs and feet to enhance the curative effect.

Sequence of the exercise: from head to toe and left to right.

☯ Opening posture

Both standing and sitting postures are viable. Let's take the standing posture as an example.

✑ Body: Total body relaxation. Stand still naturally with your eyes gently closed, tongue against the palate and lips overlapped slightly. Lower your shoulders and make your elbows loose. Separate your feet in line with your shoulders. (Picture33)

✑ Breath: Breathe naturally. Calm down. Take abdominal respiration.

✑ Meditation: Mental relaxation. Concentrate your mind on the lower dantian.

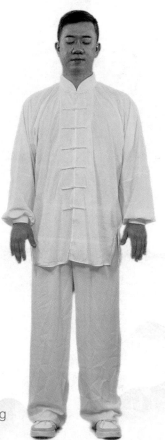

Picture33 Opening posture

附录　调养功法（英文版）

131

常见心血管病调养功法

☯ Step 1

Twist your head faceup to relax the neck

∽ Body: Twist your head backwards and repeat six times and then leftwards and rightwards four times respectively. (Picture34)

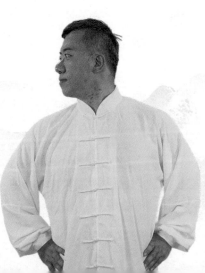

Picture34 Twist your head leftwards/rightwards

๏ Breath: Breathe naturally. Calm down. Take abdominal respiration.

๏ Meditation: Mental relaxation. Concentrate your mind on the lower dantian.

๏ Functional effect ๏

Rotating the head left and right, lifting up and down, can enhance the contraction ability of the deep and shallow muscles of the neck. And the head and neck movement has a coordinating effect on regulating the qi and blood of the zang-fu organs and the whole body. Exercise the neck muscles, help treat stiff neck and cervical spondylosis, reduce vertigo and upper limb numbness, improve neck pain and other diseases.

🌀 Step 2

Twist your shoulders to make your joints flexible

✎ Body: Twist your shoulders forwards six rounds. Rest for three seconds and then twist your shoulders backwards six rounds. Rest for three seconds and repeat four times. (Picture35)

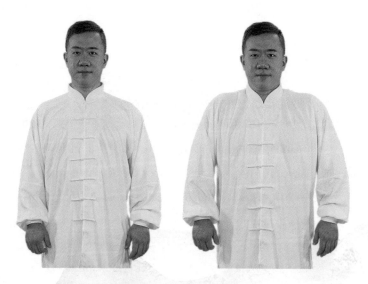

Picture35 Twist your shoulders
forwards/backwards

✐ Breath: Breathe naturally. Calm down. Take abdominal respiration.

✐ Meditation: Mental relaxation. Concentrate your mind on the lower dantian.

✐ Functional effect ✐

Twisting the shoulder, can enhance shoulder joint mobility, improve shoulder flexibility, improve local blood circulation, for the relief of shoulder periarthritis and shoulder pain discomfort has a good effect.

Step 3

Bend forwards and backwards to make your spine healthier

  Body: Raise your hands above your head and bend backwards by a small margin and keep for three seconds. Then bend forwards to touch the ground with your fingers and keep for three seconds. Next, crouch down and embrace your shoulders to keep for three seconds. Repeat four times. (From Picture36 to Picture38)

  Breath: Breathe naturally. Calm down. Take abdominal respiration.

  Meditation: Mental relaxation. Concentrate your mind on the lower dantian.

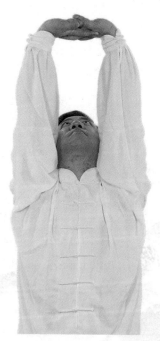

Picture36 Raise your hands above your head and bend backwards by a small margin

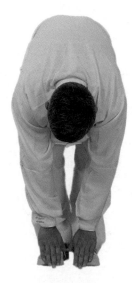
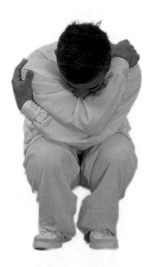

Picture37 Bend forwards to touch the ground with your fingers

Picture38 Crouch down and embrace your shoulders

❧ Functional effect ❧

This part of the movement, includes the head back, upper body back extension, forward bending, which are the main movement of the spine. The spine is the center of the whole body movement, and it is the axis of the head, neck and trunk load. Spinal exercises can not only strengthen the activities of the neck, chest, waist muscles and joints and ligaments of the cervical, thoracic and lumbar vertebrae, but also regulate the main nerves of the lower limbs (such as the sciatic nerve).

附录　调养功法（英文版）

常见心血管病调养功法

🌓 Step 4

Twist your waist to make your waist flexible

     ⌒ Body: Twist your waist counterclockwise for four rounds with your hands on your hips. Rest for three seconds and twist your waist for four rounds clockwise. Rest for three seconds and repeat three times. (Picture39)

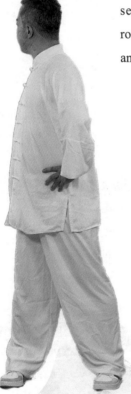

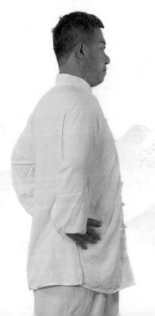

Picture39 Twist your waist with your hands on your hips

♺ Breath: Breathe naturally. Calm down. Take abdominal respiration.

♺ Meditation: Mental relaxation. Concentrate your mind on the lower dantian.

♺ Functional effect ♺

This part of the movement mainly activates the waist muscles and joints. Shaking the waist, promotes local muscle and ligament activities and plays the effect of promoting qi and blood circulation and removing blood stasis, and can improve patients' waist pain, fatigue symptoms.

常见心血管病调养功法

Closing posture

Close your eyes in tranquility. Separate your legs and put your hands alongside naturally. Breathe evenly so that you can swallow your saliva slowly. After five minutes, it is finished.